Dementia:

Management for nurses and community care workers

Key Management Skills in Nursing

Edited by Professor George Castledine and Roswyn Brown

Other titles in this series:

Managing the Acute Ward by *Jane Walton and Maggie Reeves*

Key Management Skills in Nursing
edited by
Profesor George Castledine and
Roswyn Brown

Dementia:

Management for nurses and community care workers

by
Iain B McIntosh and
Keith Woodall

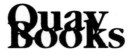

Quay Books, Mark Allen Publishing Limited
Jesses Farm, Snow Hill, Dinton, Nr Salisbury, Wilts, SP3 5HN

©Mark Allen Publishing Ltd, 1995

British Library Cataloguing-in-Publication Data
A catalogue record for this book is available from the British Library

ISBN 1-85642-117-1

Printed and bound in Great Britain by
Biddles Ltd, Guildford and King's Lynn

Contents

Chapter   Page No

Acknowledgement   vii

Foreword   ix

1   'Old timers', Alzheimer's and brain disease   1

2   Recognition and identification of dementia   9

3   Confirming the diagnosis   27

4   The nurses role   39

5   Dementia and dementia care — what are the   57
     alternatives

6   Cognitive losses and their management   71

7   Problem behaviour and its management   93

8   Sexuality and dementia   114

9   Caring for the carer   122

10   Patient safety in the community   134

Appendix   143

References   157

Index   163

Acknowledgements

Nurses are at the forefront of care in the management of patients with dementia. These patients are likely to be found in acute and long stay wards, in residential and respite care settings and the highest proportion will be found in the community. Dementia is affecting an increasing number of elderly people and, although inadequately trained, nurses will carry much of the burden of care. The topic of dementia attracts little attention in general nursing education and it is hoped that this book will help to redress this lack.

I am most appreciative of the support of Professor Mary Marshall and her staff at the Dementia Services Development Centre, University of Stirling, for the freely given access to their comprehensive data base and for permission to use material from their publications. Roswyn Brown, Principal Lecturer Postgraduate Studies in the Faculty of Health and Social Sciences at the University of Central England has been exceeding helpful with advice on the content, in proof reading and the introduction to Keith Woodall whose chapter emphasises a different perspective in nursing management of patients and carers. Data and information from the Alzheimer's Disease Society and Alzheimers Scotland/Action on Dementia is also acknowledged. My thanks are due to Staff Nurse Ann Allison who kindly supplied some of the case histories and to Nicola Ring, health visitor who assisted with proof-reading. My secretary, Pamela Littlefield has laboured steadfastly in typing this book and has accepted many unreasonable demands to meet deadlines.

As always, the unfailing support of my wife Valerie in tolerating the demands on family time, generated by production of one more book and the accompanying sudden requests for illustrations is very gratefully acknowledged.

Iain B McIntosh, BA(Hons) MBCh.B DGMRCP DRCOG
Valerie Ann McIntosh BSC (Illustrator)

Foreword

I remember, many years ago, the distress and frustration that a friend and her family experienced at the hands of their much-loved grandmother who had become prone to wandering around the house in the middle of the night. She frequently left the gas unlit on the cooker and was becoming increasingly incapable of performing even the most simple of everyday tasks which, in daily life, enable us to maintain a modicum of independence and individual dignity.

After several years of hard work and patient support from this caring family, the old lady finally died. She left behind a family unit emotionally shattered and physically exhausted, with many of their personal affairs and effects in disarray. This situation was considerably exacerbated by the fact that, unknown to them, the old lady had been secreting much of the family mail under the lid of the grand piano!

Iain McIntosh's very readable book will enable those of us who care for the demented elderly, either as lay people or as part of a multidisciplinary team in the statutory or voluntary sector, to do so in a more informed and sensitive way. Iain brings to this work a raft of experience as a general practitioner in the field of dementia care. He uses this experience to enable those engaged in this area of care to more readily identify creative ways of collaborative working, in addition to acknowledging and harnessing the contribution of a variety of agencies to the support of this deserving group of clients.

Every one of us has a vested interest in this area of care, whether we are motivated by professional altruism or self-interest (or a mixture of the two). I highly recommend that you read this book so that, together, we can all go forward in the hope of travelling at least a little way towards achieving the aim of the following statement:

'Grow old along wi' me – the best is yet to be'.

Roswyn Brown, Principal Nurse Tutor,
Postgraduate Studies

1
'Old timers' Alzheimer's and brain disease

Historical perspectives

Reference to the mental disturbances often seen in old age is first made in Greek records going back to 500 bc. In Roman times, Galen called a condition 'morosis', which he identified in people whose knowledge of letters and the arts was so totally obliterated that they could not even remember their own names. This is a description of dementia. In medieval times, the mental illness of old age was often associated with witchcraft and many demented elderly women were drowned in the ducking stool or burned at the stake. It was not until 1797 that 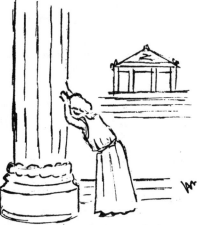 Pinel, a Frenchman, used the term 'demence' to define a patient's lack of judgment, disconnected ideas and lost faculty of mental association. Forty years later, Esquinol, another Frenchman, described dementia in clinical terms, noting that:

> *'Senile dementia is established slowly,*
> *commencing with enfeeblement of memory,*
> *actual loss of attention, the will uncertain and*
> *movements slow and impractical.'*

The link with anatomical abnormalities in the brain was made by Wilks in 1864 when he described cerebral atrophy in the wasted brain of an old man 'who had sunk mentally, into the stage of second childhood.' At the turn of the century, dementia, cerebral atrophy and distortion of microtubules in neurones in the brain cortex (neurofibrils) were firmly linked. The first paper was published by Dr Alois Alzheimer (1907), a German neurologist who gave his name to a disease which is the scourge of advanced old age and is sometimes referred to as brain failure.

Definition of the disease

Dementia exists when there is:

> *'Evidence of a decline in memory and thinking, of a degree sufficient to impair functioning in daily living, which has been present for six months or more, and is associated with an increasing impairment in emotional control, motivation and social behaviour.'*

A simpler definition is that:

> *'Dementia is a unique combination of signs and symptoms (a syndrome) resulting from global mental disturbance in an otherwise alert patient.'*

Epidemiological facts and figures

Epidemiology   is the study of the frequency, distribution and cause of disease in the general population. It is based on studies of the prevalence and incidence of the disease.

Prevalence   is the total number of patients affected by a disease in a given population at a given point in time.

Incidence differs from prevalence in that it is the number of new cases of a disease occurring in a given population in a defined time.

Dementia is very common amongst the elderly. It is a progressive illness, ultimately resulting in premature death. Overall prevalence in Scotland with a population of 5 million (1991) is 49,000 cases with a prevalence rate of 9.6 per 1000. It is estimated that there will be a 12.2% increase in the number of cases in the UK by the year 2001 (Jorm and Korten, 1987).

The prevalence of one type of dementia – Alzheimer's disease (AD) – is fast approaching epidemic proportions within the community. The number of people affected by dementia in the UK is estimated at around 750,000. AD is the most common cause of this dementia, accounting for about 50% of the cases and it affects around 500,000 older people. The current British population has 6.7% of elderly people, but this figure is increasing markedly and will not peak until the next century.

> **A nurse attached to a general practice with a list of approximately 18,000 patients might expect to find 60–80 people with definite dementia.**

It affects about 1 in 10 of those aged over 65 years and 1 in 5 of those aged over 80 years. Although many of those affected are cared for in nursing or residential homes and hospitals, the majority live in the community. Voluntary carers, often from the immediate family, carry much of the heavy burden of care but community nurses, health visitors, community psychiatric nurses and geriatric nurse visitors are all involved. In the future, they are likely to become even more involved, not only because of the increase in the population of old people, but also as a consequence of social policy which is designed to keep ill people at home for as long as possible.

The prevalence of dementia roughly doubles for every five years increase in age above the age of 65 (Jorm *et al*, 1987). Estimates from different reports suggest:

- Only 4% of demented people are under 65 years of age
- 5% are over 60 years
- 15% are over 75 years
- 22% are over 80 years
- 80% those with the disease live at home and may require community nurse support as 50% of them live on their own
- For every patient with severe dementia living in a long-stay institution, there are six living in the community
- In the case of mild to moderate dementia, for every patient living in an institution, there are 10 living in the community

It seems that about 1 in 10 to 1 in 13 of elderly people with dementia reside in hospitals and the vast majority live in the community, either at home or in NHS non-residential settings. This is an approximation of the distribution of residence in the absence of an official data base.

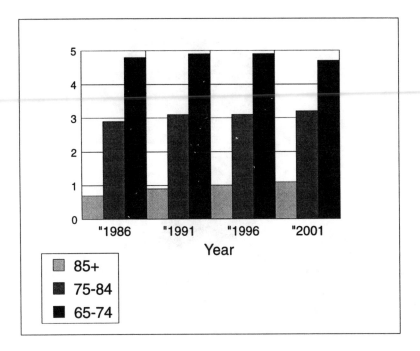

Fig 1.1 : Demographic trends (Estimate source OPCS 1991).
Population trends, 66 HMSO, London, Projections source OPCS
(1991). National population projections 1989, based Series PP2,
1017, HMSO, London.)

As the number of old people in the population rises and more
people live to a greater age, the number of cases of dementia
is expected to increase, possibly by as much as 10% in the last
decade of this century.

In dementia, brain cells die faster than they do in normal
ageing. Memory fails and the ability to carry out simple,
everyday tasks is lost. There are several types of dementia with
different causes, but their effects are much the same. The most
common is AD, which is caused by changes in the nerve cells
of the brain. The brain cells stop working properly and there is
a slow decline in mental abilities.

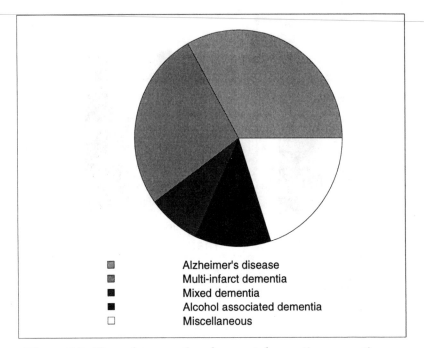

Figure 1.2: The subtypes of early onset dementia presenting to mental hospitals 1974-88*

*Source: Prevalence of Dementia 1992. Dementia Services Development Centre, Stirling (Brooks W, Whalley L).

Another type, multi-infarct dementia (MID), or arteriosclerotic dementia, accounts for 20% of cases and occurs when many tiny 'strokes' take place in the brain (Hachinsky V C *et al*, 1974). These destroy small areas of cells by cutting off the blood supply and the illness progresses in a steplike way over a period of time. Some people have both types of dementia.

Two factors are known to increase the development of AD. These are increasing age and a positive family history of dementia (Henderson, 1988). A few patients with AD show a family history of the disorder, suggesting the existence of a familial form of the illness. It has recently been recognised that there is another form of dementia, called the Cortical Lewy body type, which is responsible for a significant number of cases of dementia.

A history of previous head injury is also associated with some cases of chronic dementia and some patients with Parkinson's disease and Down's Syndrome are also more likely to develop the condition and may be more common than MID.

Prognosis

Most patients will die within four to twelve years of developing the disease and, on average, seven years after diagnosis.

The disease process

Dementia is best understood as comprising a set of symptoms caused by a variety of illnesses to which AD contributes the single most important pathology. Dementia is a syndrome resulting from disease of the brain. The condition affects the higher cortical functions, is progressive, degenerative, chronic and results in premature death.

Dementia affects brain function, destroying memory and intellect in those with the disease, thereby robbing them of personality and dignity. It is accompanied by changes in emotions, behaviour, social function and motivation. Disturbance in intellectual function occurs in clear consciousness differentiating dementia from delirium or an acute confusional state. A decline in intellectual function leads to loss of ability to perform activities of daily living such as washing, dressing and eating (Roper et al, 1990).

There is currently no cure for AD. Advances in drug therapy show promise in enhancing memory and perhaps slowing the progressive deterioration associated with the disease. Alzheimer's disease used to be called senile and pre-senile dementia. It is rare in people under 50 when it is styled AD of young onset. The disease is **not** caused by old age.

In about 5% of cases, the disease is caused by a fault in the genetic make-up, with mutations on some chromosomes.

2
Recognition and identification of dementia

The term dementia is not specific to a single underlying pathology and the condition has many different causes. The commonest cause of dementia is Alzheimer's disease (AD), often referred to as Dementia of Alzheimer's type (DAT). It accounts for around 50% of dementia cases, with cerebrovascular dementia which includes multi-infarct dementia (MID) and vascular dementias, accounting for up to 20% of cases. These conditions may also coexist. Dementia of the Cortical Lewy body type may be responsible for a significant number of cases. Some researchers consider it the second most common condition. In 5–10% of patients, rarer causes can be identified.

Dementia is an umbrella heading describing a number of pathologies (Table 2.1).

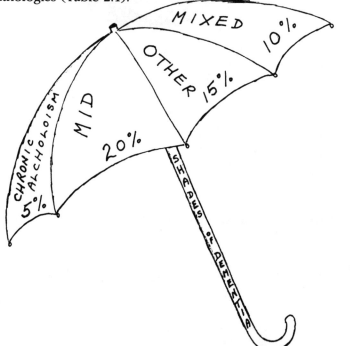

Table 2.1: Pathologies associated with dementia*

Type	%
AD	50
MID	10-20
Chronic Alcoholism	5
Lewy body type disease	15-20
Mixed MID and AD	10

AD= Alzheimer's disease
MID = Multi-infarct dementia
*Greater recognition of Cortical Lewy body type dementia may lead to revision of these figures.

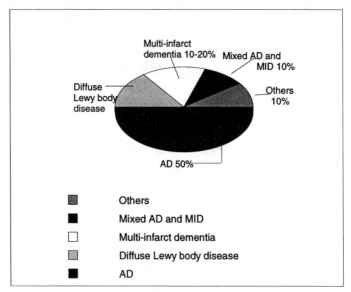

Figure 2.1: Common causes of dementia (Perry R, 1990)

Diffuse Lewy body disease (LBD)

Lewy bodies (LB) are pink-staining structures in the cytoplasm of neurones which were first described in 1912 by Lewy. These features are implicated in many cases of dementia and are particularly associated with Parkinsons disease (PD - the shaking palsy). Pathologically in PD, there is a loss of nerve cells and large numbers of Lewy bodies in the pigmented nuclei of the brain stem. Many patients suffer from both PD and AD. It has only recently become known from post-mortem examinations that a large group of dementia patients have senile plaques in their brain cortex but very few neurofibrillary tangles. Instead there are Lewy bodies. This disorder, now believed by many research workers to be the most common type of dementia after AD, has been described as dementia of the Lewy body type. The main feature differentiating patients between AD and LBD is a marked early variable symptomatology and fluctuation in cognition with changes often occurring within the space of a day and from day to day. There are often visual and auditory hallucinations. The patient may also have repeated unexplained falls or transient loss of consciousness and show mild evidence of PD, eg. rigidity, tremor, shuffling gait.

Diagnostic criteria confirming Alzheimer's Disease

- Deficits in two or more areas of cognition (cognition is the mental process by which knowledge is acquired and includes perception, reasoning and intuition)
- Progressive worsening of memory
- No disturbance of consciousness — the individual is mentally alert
- Onset between 40 and 100 years of age
- Absence of any systemic disorder
- An inevitable decline in cognitive (thinking) function and intellectual capacity

The diagnosis of AD is often made by excluding other diagnostic possibilities and relies upon finding:

- A decline in cognitive function
- An abnormal score on testing using a rating scale, e.g. many errors in memory testing

DEMENTIA: DIFFERENTIAL DIAGNOSIS CHART

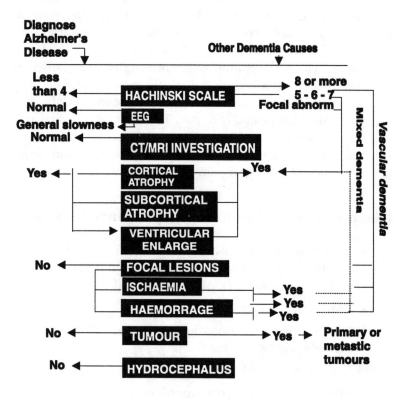

- Neuropsychological abnormalities in two different cognitive areas, e.g. memory and thinking process
- The absence of delirium

Some causes of dementia

Over 70 causes of dementia have been recognised. It is important to try and elucidate the less common causes of dementia for some of them are potentially reversible. The more common causes are :

- Primary cerebral degeneration such as AD, Parkinson's disease, dementia of the Lewy body type, Huntington's disease
- Cerebrovascular disease
- Multi-infarct dementia (cortical vascular dementia)
- Binswangers Disease (subcortical vascular dementia)
- Cerebral infections such as syphilis, meningitis and HIV infection resulting in Auto Immune Deficiency Syndrome (AIDS)
- Inflammatory systemic diseases, e.g. multiple sclerosis and systemic lupus erythematosis
- Trauma and anoxia resulting from brain injury
- Toxic causes: alcohol and drugs
- Metabolic causes: hypothyroidism, hypoglycaemia and chronic hepatic and renal problems
- Nutritional causes: vitamin B_{12} deficiency and malabsorption syndrome

A useful mnemonic for remembering the causes - **'MAMAS BITTEN DAD'**

M Multi-infarct dementia	B B$_{12}$ deficiency	D Drugs
A Alzheimer's disease	I Infection	A All other causes
M Mixed	T Trauma	D Depression
A Alcoholism	T Tumour	
S Subcortical dementia	E Endocrine	
	N Normal pressure hydrocephalus	

M ENTALLY

N AMING

H E LPS

S O M E ONE

MEM O RIZE

A N D

A I DS

Genetic causative factors   R E C ALL

There is a genetic factor in the development of AD but the mechanism of inheritance is far from clear. Nerve plaques which are characteristic in the pathology of AD are also found in adults who have Down's syndrome and it is thought that abnormalities on chromosome 21 may play a part in causation. Familial AD is a condition in which members of affected families have a higher risk of developing the symptoms than the rest of the population. Genetic link studies show an association between early-onset familial AD and chromosome 14, and between late-onset familial AD and chromosome 19 (Tobiansky, 1993). Recently, a mutation has also been found on chromosome 12.

It has been shown that ingested aluminium accumulates more in nerve cells that already contain the neurofibrillary tangles, which are the hallmark of AD. Although there does appear to be a link, the nature of the relationship has not been elucidated (Neri *et al*, 1991). Food stored in cans or cooked in aluminium pots and certain drugs, such as antacids, are sources of environmental aluminium and may produce abnormally high levels of aluminium in the blood, but this has not been substantiated.

There is no evidence to suggest that an infectious agent is implicated in the development of AD.

The course of the disease

The course is dependent upon the individual and his/her previous life experience and personality. Behaviour in those with the disease is unpredictable, with no two people exhibiting the same changes, but there are identifiable stages in the progression of the disease. These are usually considered in

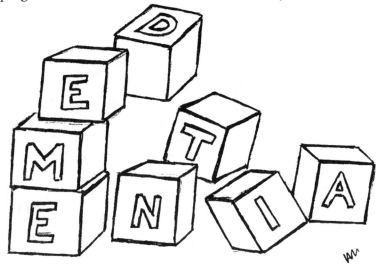

terms of early, middle and late stage dementia. A general pattern of loss has been identified and different stages can be recognised. The needs of the patient vary according to the stage of the disease and determine the service input required by the patient and carer from community and hospital care teams.

On average, patients who are affected have about nine years to live after the initial diagnosis. Efforts are now being made to detect the condition earlier. Three-quarters of GPs recently surveyed by Geriatric Medicine (1994) believed that (a) it was important to recognise AD at an early stage and (b) they were currently only dealing with the tip of the dementia iceberg. They cited the commonest current mode of presentation as problems identified by carers. With earlier diagnosis, family and community carers will be aware of the diagnosis for a longer time than in the past and will have to live longer with its implications and the stress that management of the condition generates.

Three out of four GPs find AD difficult to diagnose, but greater emphasis on training should improve this situation. Nurses involved in annual geriatric surveillance, geriatric nurse visitors and district nurses dealing with the elderly in the community are well placed to identify cases early and initiate assessment of the presenting disorder. At present, AD can only be positively confirmed at postmortem or by cerebral biopsy. Consequently it is difficult to make a firm diagnosis in the early stages of the disease. However, the disease process can be assessed by identifying disturbances in intellect, behaviour and mood. Among the most common aids to diagnosis are psychometric tests which can measure cognitive impairment. A variety of procedures may have to be used to confirm the presence of AD and exclude confounding differential diagnoses. By definition, dementia is associated with a clear consciousness. Sleepiness or drowsiness infers a more acute condition.

It should always be remembered that the progression of dementia varies considerably from person to person and that symptoms can vary from day to day, sometimes with impairment and then improvement when MID is also involved.

Early stage

The earliest sign of AD is often a degeneration of short-term memory, with patients **misplacing objects** and **forgetting** once-familiar names. This can be misconstued as evidence of benign senile forgetfulness, which accompanies ageing in many people. Objective clinical assessment can rarely detect the condition at this stage and most of those affected have no difficulty in maintaining employment and their usual social relationships. With time, however, there are occasional confusional changes, **loss of concentration and poorer attention** in reading.

Patients often recognise the changes that are affecting them and become anxious. They **deny their symptoms**, blaming them on ageing, and **work performance and social action** may be **affected**. They may become tearful, frustrated and irrational. At this stage, objective clinical testing may be valuable. Mild symptoms develop slowly with patients becoming increasingly confused and forgetting details of their own past lives. This results in a **decreased ability to handle finances** and **carry out the activities of daily living**.

Middle stage

At this stage, patients are still able to orientate themselves to place and person but denial of symptoms may become more apparent with **flattening of affect and intellectual and emotional withdrawal**. There is an inexorable decline into the development of true dementia where the person becomes totally **dependent on others** and cannot survive without assistance. Sufferers become **disorientated in time and place** and are unable to count down from twenty to one.

Patients may still be able to recall their own names and those of their immediate family and are able to feed and toilet themselves, but dressing becomes more difficult.

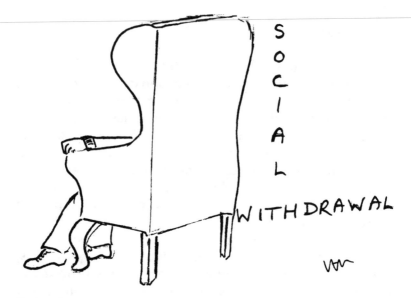

S
O
C
I
A
L

WITHDRAWAL

Late stage

As the dementia develops, patients forget the names of those closest to them, have **no recall for recent events** and have a limited recall of early experiences. Their lack of awareness may be protective. They now have difficulty in counting down from ten. Ultimately, they become **incontinent** and require assistance with most aspects of daily living.

They may begin to **wander** and turn night into day, and marked personality and emotional changes occur.They may begin to suffer **delusions** and may see their spouse as an unknown person who is a threat to them. **Obsessive, repetitive behaviour** is common and patients may become violent and demotivated. Finally, they may stop speaking, be incontinent, require feeding and **lose all basic psychomotor skills** – eventually being unable to walk. The brain is no longer able to direct the body.

Clinical features of the disease

The clinical features involve emotional, cognitive and behavioural changes.

Early stage

Emotional change features

- Shallowness of mood – swings between apathy and enthusiasm
- Poor emotional responsiveness — often low key and inappropriate
- No consideration for others — selfish and self-centred
- Depression — may be overt or masked and may not be appreciated by professional or family carer
- Anxiety — often responsible for many of the patients' behavioural and emotional reactions

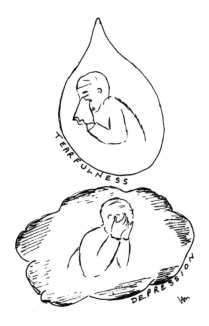

Cognitive changes

- Short-term memory impairment
- Difficulty in recalling new information
- Thinking becomes inflexible
- Repetitive speech and perseverance of thoughts and activities

Behavioural changes

- Social withdrawal
- Difficulty in carrying out activities of daily living
- Inappropriate social behaviour
- Self-neglect
- Emotional disinhibition
- Disorientation — in terms of time initially, then relating to place and, finally, to people

Case history

Mrs P had been a school headmistress for many years, and had rather a dominant personality. At home, where she had lived with a sister for ten years, she had always been a little eccentric. A great reader, she had recently lost interest in her books and began to make mistakes in the household finances. At first, she laughed at these, but had now become so secretive about the errors that the sister was never allowed to see the bills. Final demands for unpaid bills began to appear.

When Mrs P was questioned by the sister, she became physically and verbally aggressive. Gradually, her loss of memory for recent events became more apparent. She had mood swings between euphoric and, at other times, tearful states. She grew increasingly garrulous and neglectful of her dress and personal hygiene. She began wandering away from the house along the

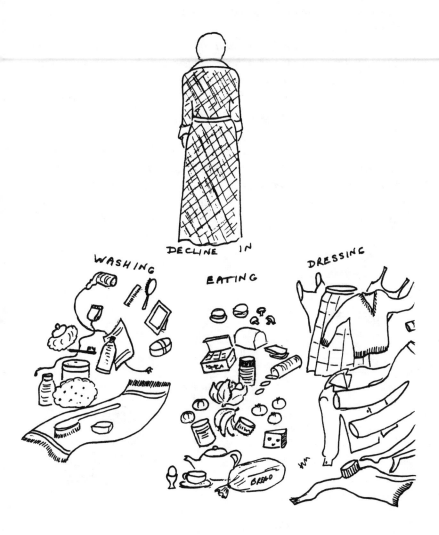

street and was obviously disorientated in time and place when brought back.

The sister had tolerated what she considered merely selfish and very eccentric behaviour for nearly two years before increasing violence drove her to seek medical help.

Mrs P was assessed by her GP who referred her for psycho-geriatric appraisal. A diagnosis of probable AD was made after all investigations had proved negative. Aware of the diagnosis and prognosis, the sister sought additional home help and a programme of respite care was organised to help her carry some of the burden. A rare episode of acute agitation was treated with thioridazine when it occurred, and she stayed within community care.

Middle stages

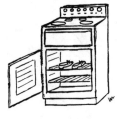
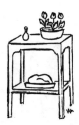
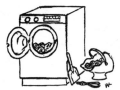

Emotional changes

- Irritability and hostility
- Aggression

Cognitive changes

- Receptive and expressive dysphasia
- Disordered and fragmented speech

- Ideas of persecution
- Delusions
- Auditory and visual hallucinations

Behavioural changes

- Wandering and restlessness
- Turning night into day
- Aggression and violence

Later stages

In the later stages there may be:

- Weight loss
- Malnutrition
- Self-neglect
- Bradykinesia (slowing of normal movement)
- Tremor
- Incontinence of urine and faeces
- Rigidity of muscles and body
- Instability and, ultimately, immobility

Case history

Mr Jones suffered from Parkinsonism for six years and, gradually, it robbed him of his mobility. He became very fearful, obsessed with his body functions and began to have difficulties in remembering words. This, together with a slowing of his speed of enunciation and intensity of vocalisation created major communication problems for him and his carer. His nights became very disturbed and, finally, he started to climb out of bed and urinate in a corner of the bedroom. Formerly, a demure, reticent man, he began to sexually expose himself on his rare public appearances. Clinical and other investigations supported a diagnosis of dementia associated with Parkinson's disease. Initially, efforts were made to provide further carer support by community staff, but his condition deteriorated. He stopped eating and drinking of his own motivation, became incontinent of urine and was eventually admitted to a long-care psychogeriatric ward. Drug efforts to control the urinary incontinence had proved valueless and the constant changing of personal and bed linen, aggravated by the disruptive behaviour proved too much for his wife's health and she succumbed to illness and short-term hospital admission.

Points to remember

- Dementia of the Alzheimer's type usually presents with an insidious onset
- The onset can occur over months or years, can be stable for a while and then become progressive
- If multi-infarct dementia, progression is usually stepwise
- Alertness is normal
- Orientation is usually disturbed for time and place but may be normal
- Memory is impaired for recent times
- Thoughts are slowed with a reduction in interest
- There is often associated depression which may respond to drug therapy
- Perception may be normal but hallucinations often occur
- Emotions are shallow, labile and apathetic
- Sleep is often disturbed with nocturnal wandering or nocturnal confusion

- There are often and, ultimately, personality changes with catastrophic reactions

It can be helpful to consider the stages as mild, moderate and severe, with people in the last category probably receiving nursing care within a nursing home or hospital.

Table 2.2: Diagnosis chart

	DEMENTIA	DELIRIUM	DEPRESSION
1. Onset	Insidious	Acute	Gradual
2. Duration	Months/years	Hours/days/ ??weeks	Weeks or months
3. Course	Stable and progressive (unless MID – usually stepwise)	Flucuates – worse at night Lucid periods	Usually worse in morning, improves as the day goes on
4. Alertness	Usually normal	Fluctuates	Normal
5. Orientation	**May** be normal – usually impaired for time and place	Always impaired Time Place Person	Usually normal
6. Memory	Impaired recent and sometimes remote memory	Recent impaired	Recent may be impaired Remote intact
7. Thoughts	Slowed Reduced interests Perseverate	Often paranoid and grandiose, ? bizarre ideas topics, ? paranoid	Usually slowed, preoccupied sad and hopeless

	DEMENTIA	DELIRIUM	DEPRESSION
8. Perception	? Normal Hallucinations occur in 30–40% (often visual)	Visual and auditory hallucinations common	20% have mood congruent auditory hallucinations
9. Emotions	Shallow, apathetic, labile, ?irritable, careless	Irritable Aggressive Fearful	Flat, unresponsive or sad and fearful. May be imitable
10. Sleep	Often disturbed. Nocturnal wandering common, nocturnal confusion	Nocturnal confusion	Early morning wakening
11. Other features		Other physical disease may not be obvious	? past history of mood disorder

Source: Dementia touches everyone - a training guide for general practitioners, McLennan, Murdoch, Mcintosh

3
Confirming the diagnosis

Differential diagnosis

Differential diagnosis is very important in dementia because the symptoms may be caused by other conditions which may be reversible if diagnosed early enough. Scientists in the USA have developed a Diagnostic and Statistical Manual of Mental Disorders (DSM 111(R). It sets out criteria which aid the recognition of dementias.

Criteria for the diagnosis of AD

* Dementia
  Mild Work or social activities are significantly impaired but capacity for independent living remains, with personal hygiene and judgment intact
  Moderate Independent living is hazardous and some degree of supervision is necessary
  Severe Activities of daily living are so impaired that continual supervision is required. Patients are unable to maintain personal hygiene and may be incoherent or mute
* Insidious onset with a generally progressive deteriorating course
* Exclusion of all other specific causes of dementia

Primary AD can present as delirium, delusions and depression, or be uncomplicated. These are complicating factors in diagnosis that should be constantly kept in mind.

Several rating scales have been developed to aid diagnosis. A commonly used rating scale is the Mini-Mental State

Examination (MMSE) or an alternative version called the Abbreviated Mental Test (AMT). A third is Alzheimer's Disease Assessment Scale (ADAS) which is specifically designed for use with AD patients. It assesses cognitive performance and behaviour and involves interviews with the carer. Activities of daily living scales are also used, such as the Instrumental Activities of Daily Living and the BARTHEL Index. High scores suggest a high degree of impairment. There are several other commonly used scales. Some of these are complex and many are time-consuming (see Appendix for examples).

Common confounding causes of dementia

The diagnosis of dementia can be confused with that of delirium and depression. However, dementia has an insidious onset, whereas the onset of delirium is usually acute and that of depression is gradual. Unfortunately, demented patients can also suffer from depression and some dementing symptoms are also features of acute delirium. Table 3.1 lists the features which differentiate the disorders.

Table 3.1: Features differentiating dementia, delirium and depression

		Depression (Pseudodementia)	Dementia
History	Onset	dated accurately	vague
	Progression	can be rapid	slowly progressive
	Length of symptoms	short duration	long duration
	Family	aware of disabilities early on	unaware of disability until later
Symptomatology	Memory loss	patients complain of loss	patients rarely complain of loss
	Disability	emphasise disability	hide disability
	Time	worse in the morming	confusion worse in the evening
Investigations			
Computed tomography		scant evidence of atrophy	cerebral atrophy and ventricular enlargement
Electroencephalogram		usually normal	pronounced slow activity
Single photon emission tomography		blood flow patterns normal	parieto-temporal and frontal abnormalities

The reversible causes of dementia are sometimes known as pseudodementia and it is very important to recognise them so that treatment may be instituted. There are many causes of acute confusion (Table 3.2).

Table 3.2: Causes of acute confusion

Infection	Chest infections and urinary tract infections are frequent causes
Toxic reactions	Commonly occur as a result of drug medication, alcohol addiction, the withdrawal of medication or drug interactions
Electrolyte imbalance	Occurs as a result of disturbance in potassium, sodium and water in the body
Arterial oxygen insufficiency	Results from decreased efficiency of the cardiovascular system, e.g. after myocardial infarction
Cerebral arterial disturbance	Following stroke
Hormonal and metabolic disturbance	Occurs in thyroid disorders, such as myxoedema or hypothyroidism. Also occurs with hypoglycaemia or hyperglycaemiain diabetes and in renal failure or uraemia
Chronic malnutrition	Often occurs in elderly people living alone
Skull injury	E.g. resulting from subdural haematomas
Brain disorders	Tumour and hydrocephalus are common causes

Source: Dementia troubles everyone — a training guide for general practitioners, McLennan, Murdoch and McIntosh

Of all patients apparently suffering from dementia, perhaps 10% will have a possibly reversible cause, such as an acute confusional state. Others will have depression which may be treatable.

Depression

Between 15 and 20% of people aged over 65 years suffer from a depressive disorder and this diagnosis must be kept firmly in mind when treating patients with possible dementia. Unfortunately, some patients with dementia also suffer from depression and it can be difficult to separate the two. The use of rating scales such as the Hamilton Depression Rating Scale (see Appendix) can aid differentiation.

Toxic confusional states, depression and other physical disorders often occur in dementing patients and complicate diagnosis; it is important to unearth alternative causes so that appropriate treatment can be instituted to improve mental and physical states. Ability to differentiate between the types of dementia will be important when drug management becomes established. Faced with decisions regarding diagnosis, it is useful to remember:

1   Alzheimer's disease is gradual in onset and usually occurs in people over 45 years of age. It is progressive with global deterioration.

2   Multi-infarct dementia has an onset from the age of 55 years onwards; it often occurs suddenly with localising neurological signs such as transient ischaemic attacks. Past history often reveals cardiovascular problems. It is thought to be more prevalent in men than women and the progression often shows a stepwise decline in skills and emotions and intermittent personality changes.

3   In Lewy body-type dementia, there is usually some evidence of arterial vascular disease elsewhere and localised neurological signs.

4   Vitamin B12 deficiency: this is usually associated with anaemia and changes in behaviour are obvious. It can also be associated with low folic acid levels and there may be sensory nerve changes in the legs and arms.

5   Hypothyroidism: a flagrant myxoedema is now relatively rare. Many older women and a few older

men suffer from hypothyroidism; however, this is not obvious without a blood test.

6   Tumour: primary and secondary tumours are common in the elderly.

Investigations aiding diagnosis

The existence of **some of these conditions can be confirmed from blood investigations**. It may fall to the attending nurse to confirm that blood investigations have been instigated and completed (McIntosh, 1990). There should be recent notes in the patient's records which should include:

- A full blood count
- Vitamin B_{12} and folate levels
- Thyroid function tests
- Urea and electrolytes
- Liver function tests
- Blood glucose
- Calcium levels

These are all useful screening tools which help to rule out treatable causes of dementia. The advent of annual GP geriatric assessment of all those over 75 years of age, has provided an opportunity to screen for dementia and other diseases. A comprehensive check list of physical, mental, functional and sonal status has proved useful and has been welcomed by patients (McIntosh, 1990 and 1993; Wilkinson, (1995). When other diagnostic exclusions have been considered and dealt with in the community, assessment of care needs can be initiated.

Functional capacity

The needs of the patient which have to be considered

Is the patient:
- Coping with routine tasks
- Lacking in self-care
- Showing emotional changes of anxiety, depression, other memory lapses
- Safe in the confines of his/her environment
- Disorientated in time and place

The ability to carry out activities of daily living (ADL) are crucial if the patient is to continue in the home setting. This often determines the need for placement in residential or nursing homes, or long-stay institutions. These include:
- Continence
- Dressing
- Self-care
- Home safety
- Financial arrangements
- Cooking skills
- Self-nutrition and shopping
- Social contacts

What are **the carers' needs** and are they coping?
- Is their physical and mental health sound?
- Are they sleeping well and do they have any free time?
- Is there a bridge between their needs and the services provided?

- Should additional members of the caring team be involved?

- Is there good communication between the members of the caring team who are currently involved?

Nurses should be involved in the general elements of history taking and assessment and may, in the community, be expected to operate rating scales and activities of daily living scales (McIntosh, 1990). Once all the material has been accumulated, a case conference of the primary care team members should, ideally, be set up in conjunction with the social work care manager to review the data on patient and carer. At this conference, a comprehensive treatment and management plan should be agreed. This may take time and the immediate input is likely to depend on the nurse's personal skills in dealing with the current situation.

Support services vary from area to area but it is important for the nurse to be aware of what can be made available (see diagram p35).

Further aids to diagnosis

The earlier the disease can be detected and diagnosed, the sooner palliative management can be initiated (McIntosh, 1993). Information obtained from rating scales and structured diagnostic interviews can be of great value in the screening exercise. Rating scales often have limited value but are popular and, if short, can be easily utilised in the primary care setting. As dementia consists of disturbance of intellect, behaviour and mood, all three can be assessed, and scales are of help, not only in the initial diagnosis but also in monitoring the progression of the illness. However, they remain only aids in assisting with the diagnosis and should be used in conjunction with clinical appraisal and judgment. Key items which appear to discriminate people with dementia relate to memory and orientation (Orrell, 1992).

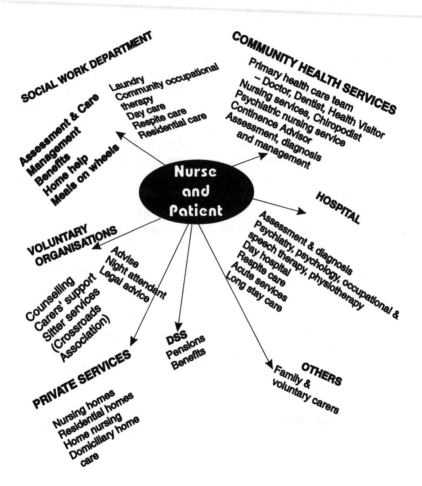

Figure 3.1: Care associations

Psychometric tests are commonly used to measure cognitive impairment. A commonly used example of a rating scale is the (**MMSE**, Folstein, 1975) which is a short and easily administered quantitative test (see appendix for illustration of MMSE). Its value in establishing the absence or presence of cognitive impairment has been validated (Tombaugh, 1992). A score of less than 25 as a consistent response makes a diagnosis of AD probable. A score below 13 on the 30 point scale is predictive as 87% of people with dementia score below 23 points on the MMSE. Shorter versions, such as the Abbreviated Mental Test Scale (**AMTS**) are also used, although their brevity have limitations. However, they may point the way towards early recognition of dementia. The MMSE includes questions on instant recall, short-term memory, series of fractions and reverse spelling (Iliffe, 1994). The (AMTS) is a 10-item test, primarily assessing orientation, although it also considers memory, recognition of persons, calculation and attention.

A rating scale to differentiate between AD and vascular dementia (VAD) has been developed and is used by physicians, but it does not differentiate between a mixed AD and VAD (Hachinsky, 1974) – see appendix.

The **ADAS** was specifically designed for use with AD patients (Rosen, 1984). It is usually rated by the physician or the psychologist and takes about ten minutes to do. The Cambridge examination for mental disorders of the elderly (CAMDEX) is another frequently used aid.

The **Blessed Dementia Scale** measures aspects of daily life, such as competence in coping with household chores, money and shopping lists (Blessed, 1968).

Physical tests are also of value and include activities of daily living scales, such as Instrumental Activities of Daily Living which can be measured IADL scale (Lawton, 1969). High scores suggest a higher degree of impairment. One other useful assessment protocol which is often used in screening, is the

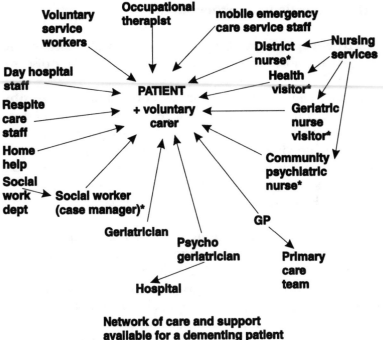

Voluntary service workers

Occupational therapist

mobile emergency care service staff

District nurse*

Nursing services

Day hospital staff

PATIENT

Health visitor*

Respite care staff

+ voluntary carer

Geriatric nurse visitor*

Home help

Social work dept

Social worker (case manager)*

Community psychiatric nurse*

Geriatrician

Psycho geriatrician

GP

Primary care team

Hospital

Network of care and support available for a dementing patient living in the community

*possible key worker

Clifton Assessment Procedure for the Elderly (CAPE) (Pattie, 1980) which can be rated by nurses and takes 25 to 30 minutes to do. Rating general dependency is valuable and the BARTHEL Index is often used – see Appendix.

Depression must be considered in the differential diagnosis. In depression monitoring, the **Hamilton Depression Rating Scale** is useful and **Brief Assessment Schedule Depression Cards** (BASDEC) can provide quick scoring guides to the existence of depression in elderly people (Adshead, 1992; Hamilton, 1960).

Other investigative procedures

Electroencephalography (EEG) is occasionally used where there is a possibility that epilepsy may be a feature of the disease.

Currently, new techniques such as **computed tomography** (CT) scan, a non-invasive imaging technique that can produce cross-sectional images of the brain by using multiple X-ray images, is proving of value. It can detect enlargement of the ventricles in the brain and widening of the sulci – possible indications of degenerative brain disease. The technique is also useful in detecting brain tumours and infarcts.

Magnetic resonance imaging (MRI), although only available in a limited number of areas in the UK, does effectively detect AD changes in the brain at an early stage. A new technique, **positron emission tomography** (PET), can show a characteristic profile for AD in comparison with other types of dementia. It can identify a global reduction in cerebral metabolism, which is particularly prominent in the parietal and temporal lobes of AD patients, and it may well be that this technique will be increasingly used in the future. PET measures the function of brain cells by analysing the brain's ability to utilise glucose. In AD, the affected parts of the brain are areas of non-function.

Single photon emission computed tomography (SPECT) employs a radioactive labelled marker to produce images of blood flow in the brain. In AD there is reduced cerebral blood flow, whereas in infarction there is complete absence of blood from the area because of tissue death.

4
The nurse's role

Nursing assessment

The full assessment procedure may require several visits and involve other members of the multi-disciplinary care team as well as the nurse.

In the foreseeable future, it would appear that the overall care and support of those with dementia will be given by doctors, nurses and other paramedics, and their role will continue to be vital until drug therapy can either bring cure or greatly alleviate the effects of the disease. Input will vary depending on whether the nurse is working in the community on the district, as a community psychiatric nurse, community-liaison nurse or in a nursing home or specialist unit.

Psychiatric nurses have a role in mental health care which has changed rapidly over the last decade. Although hospital based, they now have an expanding work commitment within the community. In the past their work with demented patients was associated with the provision of long-term care in long-stay institutions. These nurses have specialist skills in caring for individuals with mental health problems. In response to the concept of patient care within the community, psychiatric nurses are now working in long-stay units, day hospitals, memory clinics and in nursing homes for the mentally disabled within the private sector.

The number of **community psychiatric nurses** is likely to increase further, creating many new opportunities and alternatives in care provision for the demented, thus benefiting patients and carers. Many have a specialist remit to care for patients living at home and their work load may be predominantly with the dementing elderly. They can provide support and help to reduce the stress on the patient, the caring family and on other nurses from the primary care team (Rawlinson, 1992).

Primary care team nurses are traditionally part of the primary care team and are often attached to general medical practices or directly employed by fund-holding doctors who buy in their services. This association facilitates liaison between members of the team — a particularly important element of good home care for dementing people.

Health visitors and district nurses are key workers in primary care and may act as team leaders in some situations. Some practices also have geriatric nurse visitors who are likely to have many contacts with dementing patients on the practice list (McIntosh 1990). The initiation of annual geriatric screening has resulted in many health visitors and nurses developing special interests and skills in dementia care (McIntosh, 1993; Wilkinson, 1995), thus they are ideally placed to make early identification of new patients with dementia and for monitoring progress of established cases.

The differing and separate roles of the health visitor and the district nurse will ensure that there are specific benefits to the dementing patient, which can only be provided by that particular health care professional. For example, the district nurse as a provider of nursing intervention and the health visitor as a promotor of good health. However, there are some areas of service-delivery which both professionals can provide. These include assessment and monitoring, eg. in incontinence, acting as a resource by referring the patient to social work departments and providing support and counselling, particularly to carers.

In practice, the nurse primarily responsible for an individual patient will be dictated by circumstances. The professional, whether health visitor or district nurse, with the most appropriate skills will deliver the necessary care at the time when it is needed. Good communication between the health visitor and the district nurse is vital for effective management.

Community nurses (district nurses) are usually attached to general practices and are responsible for nursing duties within the community. Initially, they may become involved if there are physical frailties, loss of mobility, incontinence and behavioural problems with a dementing patient.

Geriatric health nurse visitors have been attached to some general practices and are frequently responsible for carrying out much of the annual geriatric assessment contractually required from GPs. In many cases, they visit the elderly on a quarterly, six-monthly or annual basis and many are skilled at completing assessment protocols, dementia and depression rating scales in the elderly population. They pay particular attention to the competence of the individual in caring for him/herself and whether there are problems developing, eg. malnutrition or hypothermia (McIntosh, 1988).

Social work care managers are social workers appointed by the local authority to assess the individual's needs before planning any intervention. They are the fund holders and when an assessment has been completed the care manager will contact service providers with respect to setting up home help, Meals on Wheels and mobile emergency care. Alternatively, they may approach residential or nursing home managers or the local nursing team for placement and assistance. The care manager is responsible for monitoring the ongoing package of care which can be provided by voluntary, NHS and/or private agencies.

Clinical nurse specialists can now be found in day hospitals, psychogeriatric day hospitals, respite care units, geriatric wards and geriatric rehabilitation units. These professionals have developed additional skills in the treatment of demented patients. Although many of the problems created by the dementing are easier to contain within hospital and nursing homes, institutionalisation creates new problems which require different types of management.

Occupational therapists are attached to some districts and are involved in the assessment of activities of daily living needs, and are responsible for ensuring that an appropriate home environment is available. They play a valuable role in reality orientation and reminiscence therapies.

Irrespective of roles, all members of the **care team** have as their **objectives**: the improvement of the quality of patient care; the provision of optimal support for patient and carer and the

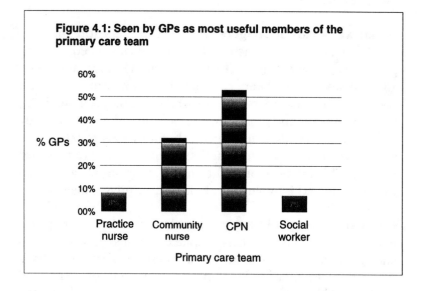

Figure 4.1: Seen by GPs as most useful members of the primary care team

reduction of stress in the carer until such time as admission to a long-stay unit becomes necessary.

Assessment

A comprehensive assessment can rarely be completed in one visit and ongoing re-assessments are required to map the progression of dementia. By structuring the assessment and resorting to the carer-using protocols and questionnaires, it is easier to cover all the essential points necessary for adequate management.

Assessment goals

- Diagnose dementing illness
- Discriminate between types of dementia
- Measure the change and the progressive of the illness
- Determine the level of functioning
- Determine the effectiveness of carer intervention

The nursing process

Irrespective of environment, the framework for the practice of nursing has been well established since the early 1980s. It has been based on a problem-solving system – the nursing process – with an application in four stages committed to delivery of care in the form of:

- Assessment
- Planning
- Intervention
- Evaluation

The application of this process has generated a systematic approach to nursing and the main functions are:

- Clinical activities involving assessment, treatment and monitoring
- Psychosocial activities involving the establishment and exploitation of the therapeutic relationship
- Environmental assessment and its manipulation where necessary
- Liaison with other members of the primary care and mental health teams, and those responsible for implementing the Community Care Act, and, of

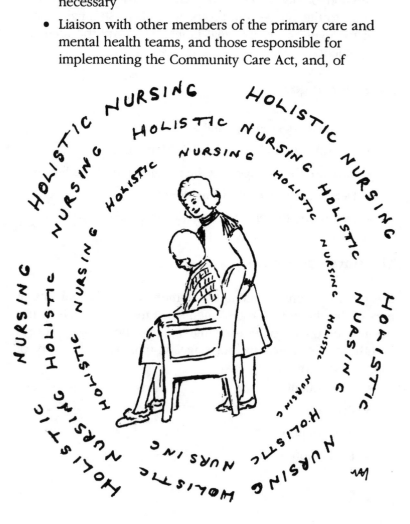

particular importance in the case of dementia, liaison with the carer.

Nursing staff are likely to continue to make a major contribution in supporting the demented and their carers, if for no other reason than that medical science has, as yet, little to offer in terms of treatment.
The main problems of dementing and demented patients are their inability to carry out activities of daily living. This means that, in many instances, the nurse will have a primary role to play. It may be that in the guise of geriatric nurse visitor in a rural setting, or as a practice nurse, he or she will retain the principal role. The nursing profession will be involved with patients and relatives in the home setting, and within day hospitals and inpatient facilities.

The nurse role

The role is twofold:

1 To maintain patients' independence at the maximum level of individual ability

2 To provide support for patients and relatives

The provisions of the National Health Service and Community Care Act 1990 establish a clear principle that dementing patients and the demented should be kept in their own homes for as long as possible.
Nursing, with its holistic, global and person-centred approach to care, should take the lead in maintaining the highest quality of life for dementia sufferers and their carers. In the past, nursing care has tended to focus on maximising the functional ability of the patient and helping carers to cope with the results of the disease process – **a biomedical model**. This provides a rather passive and purely palliative role. Undoubtedly, good nursing based on this model can relieve some of the problems

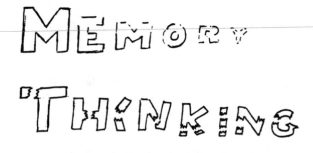

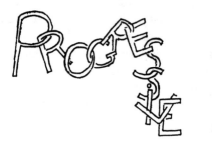

associated with dementia, especially those of a behavioural nature, such as wandering or restlessness. A much wider approach, however, is required to deal with the multiplicity of cognitive, emotional, behavioural and social problems that are associated with the dementing process (Watkins, 1988).

A viewpoint based on accepting confused behaviour as an understandable reaction of the sufferer to the stresses of powerlessness, loss of control and social isolation, which can affect the dementia sufferer, has to be adopted by those nursing such patients.

A proliferation of techniques, such as reality orientation, validation therapy, reminiscence therapy, resolution therapy and life reviews (see chapter 6) has been embraced by nurses working within this field in the last few years (Janssen, 1988). The techniques help to maintain social skills and provide additional sensory stimulation and socialisation in individuals who are often isolated in their own homes. This is an endeavour to improve and maintain existing cognitive abilities.

An increasing number of people with dementia will have to be cared for within the community or in nursing homes. Currently, many demented patients have less than ideal community support, with as many as 30% having no access to specialist dementia services. Their mental state often deprives them of an understanding of their own needs and many carers are still reluctant to take up the facilities and support offered by social services and to claim attendance allowances.

Nurses are often the first point of contact with the individual in the early stage of dementia and, because of the physical decline associated with the disease, are likely to have a long, continuous and intense relationship with these patients. This has the advantage of providing opportunities to implement some of the new therapies. Input has to be of an holistic nature with a global approach but should also remain family-centred and focused on the individual — **a holistic model.**

The aim is the provision of a flexible service which can be nurse-led. It has to be used in combination with a systematic assessment and problem-solving approach, either as the nurse involved in annual geriatric surveillance, in a community screening exercise for dementia, or as a practice nurse or a clinical nurse specialist. Potentially, all are in a position to undertake preliminary diagnostic assessments. With education and practice, their skills are ideal for the development of nursing practice within dementia services.

It is well recognised that, currently, the nurse's role in giving information to carers and promoting carers' health with counselling and support is underdeveloped. Their input can be vital in a household where there is a demented patient. Ideally, the needs and interest of all groups have to be considered (Masterson, 1993).

All nurses dealing with demented patients have the potential to develop positive and optimistic views with regard to dementia and the capacity of people suffering from dementia to live at ease with their impairment. These personal beliefs have to be conveyed to the patients. There has to be the recognition that a shift from physical care work to

psychotherapeutic care work is necessary, a bridge that some caring, conscientious nurses find difficult to cross. Nurses who work in this field need to acknowledge that their contribution to care work extends beyond professional physical actions and includes their own behaviour, emotions and responses. The nurse should develop the ability and the willingness to confront and appreciate the devastation and trauma that dementia inflicts on the sufferer. It is crucial to try to understand the patient's experience and comprehension of what has happened to him/her.

Health professionals, especially nurses, can expect to manage an increasing number of cases of dementia and confusion (Evers, 1982). There is still a common impression that, once marked mental deterioration sets in, there is little that can be done for an individual other than to provide basic care. This view is not supported by research findings.

There has been a tendency for nursing staff to regard their care priority as a physical rather than a psychosocial interaction with restorative activities (Brooking, 1986). In one study (Armstrong and Esther, 1986), it was found that there were low levels of staff/patient communication, with nurses interacting significantly less with confused patients than with lucid patients. Nurses must guard against responding in a qualitatively different way to confused and demented patients in comparison with those who have good understanding. Brown (1989) found that task-centred nurses tended to communicate with patients only on those occasions when a physical nursing procedure was being carried out. In situations where the patient did not speak English or was not *compos mentis*, there was little communication at all.

People with dementia have the same range of needs as other members of the community and other patients. Their needs for security and physical care are critical. So too, however, are needs to maintain social relationships and opportunities for expressions of their individuality and sense of self-worth. Attitudes to care are vitally important in terms of satisfactory outcome of care-giving procedures. Woods has outlined several criteria (Woods, 1987). These are:

1 Dementia sufferers should be accorded full respect and dignity

2 They should be treated appropriately for their actual age

3 They should be helped to participate in good social relationships with the ordinary community

Frames of reference

To achieve these goals, nurses need to have an adequate knowledge of dementia and the psychological and other approaches that can be used in individualised care.

Before tackling the care plan, nurses should ask themselves, 'What is the personal frame of reference?' If the first thought is 'Yet another case of Alzheimer's' then the frame of reference is medical. If, however, they see a person struggling with memory loss and psychological disturbance beyond their ability to cope, as well as a person with professional training and specialist skills who has carried a suitcase of life's experiences, then the frame of reference will be one of understanding. If only psychological, physical deficits and problems, and the need for systematic assessment are seen, then the frame of reference may be manipulative and interventionist.

Ideally, in caring for dementing patients, one needs a mental set of understanding and a view of the patient as someone who has lost everyday faculties which allow them to carry out activities of daily living, is losing control over themselves and, ultimately, the knowledge of who or what they are.

One useful basis for understanding is given by Kitwood (1993). He offers the equation:

$$d = p+b+h+ni+sp$$

where d = dementia, p = personality, b = biography, h = physical health, ni = neurological impairment and sp = social psychology.

Personality refers to the temperament of each individual and his/her life's experience.

Biography refers to what has happened to the person throughout his /her life in terms of relationships, opportunities and deprivations.

Physical health is obviously important, if only to exclude other causes of confusion and to confirm that problem behaviours may be evidence that the patient is suffering from discomfort, pain or a physical cause which can be alleviated.

Neurological impairment relates to brain damage and the interference with neurotransmitter mechanisms, and finally

Social psychology encompasses what is happening to a patient moment by moment in everyday life – a domain that relates to 'person-hood'.

If the focus is primarily on neurological impairment then an 'us' and 'them' situation can be created. We have the brains and the skills and are rational and responsive; they simply have problems in behaviours and react with irrational responses.

Good dementia management depends upon an understanding attitude and it is important for a nurse not to carry in the 'personal suitcase' a 'them and us' attitude (Kitwood, 1993), viewing the dementia sufferer as unsound of mind, neurologically impaired, brain damaged or mentally deficient and assuming that, as a professional, he/she is normal.

Intervention by the professional brings its own problems. Any person who would care for dementing patients and their carers must be prepared to deal with their own self-defeating patterns of behaviour before tackling the problem. A 'therapeutic' awareness of this kind should be a central part of caring for dementia sufferers. The presence of dementia raises deep questions about what it means to suffer from the disease and its effect on the affected person. The disease appears to take the 'self' away and carers must strive to leave the person involved with status and self-respect.

Management of dementia

This involves assessing the needs of dementia sufferers and their carers and designing interventions that will increase independent functioning. This is based on individual care to specifically address the needs of dementia sufferers in the broadest sense, identifying their resources and abilities. The process then permits a care plan to be drawn up, keeping in mind specific goals or targets to be achieved by the patient. This approach has been evaluated by Brody *et al*, (1974). It has been proved successful in terms of showing improvements in the areas tackled directly by care-giving programmes, and even after long-term follow-up there was a reported 30% success rate in goal-plan achievement (Barraclough, 1986).

The whole process involves consideration of patient, family and environment (see figure 4.2). The needs assessment stage is crucial and often little time is devoted to it, with health care professionals launching immediately into therapeutic intervention. A complete picture of patient function, considering the patient's present and past state of total wellbeing, is essential and should involve a review of the medical assessment of the sufferer and the carer, taking into account:

1   Family and social networks

2   Clear life-cycle of those concerned

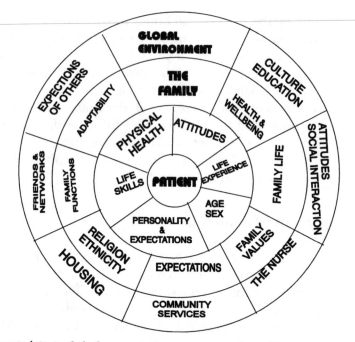

Figure 4.2: A global approach – assessing the patient and family and environment

3   Social and economic situation

4   Their current functioning status

5   Perceived problems and their immediacy

In the early stages of dementia, the individual may be functioning quite well outside the home, but if the diagnosis is suspected it is best to carry out this interview in the home environment where the carer can also be interviewed. Carr and Marshall (1993) from the Dementia Services Development Centre call for a more thoughtful approach to defining needs as there are different stages in the progression of the dementia. They suggest the need for a profile which provides a picture in terms of characteristics such as physical problems, sociability, self-care skills, coexisting psychiatric problems, nursing dependency and behaviour. Equipped with such a picture, the health care professional can then define and systematise the patient's needs

The nursing care of patients with dementia is focused on maximising the functional ability of the patient and helping care-givers to cope with illness. Nursing intervention should focus on strategies for dealing with problems involving verbal and non-verbal communication, physical functioning, perceptional and motor difficulties, memory loss and social isolation. Good individualised care can be accomplished by knowing the patient's previous interests and occupations, and allowing family involvement. The family's perspective and objectives must be considered if an optimal standard of care is to be attained for each patient. Family input needs to be sought as a vital aspect of mutual decision-making regarding care (see global assessment diagram, figure 4.2).

Management models

Two main models have been utilised in supporting patients and their carers, one patient-orientated and the other care-giver orientated; both have a problem-solving approach. It is difficult to separate the two strategies. Although a trained nurse can rapidly assess a patient's nursing requirements using an activities of daily living model, it is more difficult to identify priority needs for the care-giver and recourse may be made to a model of care such as that for dementia stress management.

A feature of almost all psychological intervention is the assumption that a person can acquire new information and learn new skills, the very area in which dementia sufferers are most impaired. However, research has shown that dementia sufferers are able to learn new information and that their behaviour can change with appropriate training, (although at a slower rate; see Chapter 10).

There are four means of learning: classical conditioning, operant learning, motor learning and verbal learning. All of

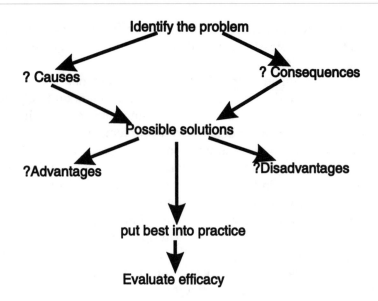

Figure 4.3: Dementia Management Flow Chart

these have been shown to be preserved in dementia, at least in the early and middle stages. The ultimate aim in care is to maximise self-care. This in itself can create a nursing problem as it often takes longer to encourage a person to do a task than for the nurse to do it for the patient. Allowing time for the dementing patient to comply with instructions and perform functions can be a difficult adaptive process for time-constrained nurses, who are trained to provide the immediate response so often required in physical features of other nursing disciplines. The main objective is to re-institute behaviours that may have existed in the past and which may have been lost. This is, however, dependent on some basic skills remaining intact.

A structured assessment plan

The following list of the individuals activities of daily living can be used to structure the assessment and planning of care:

- Maintaining a safe environment (involves memory and orientation)
- Communication
- Eating and drinking skills
- Urinary and faecal control
- Hygiene standards
- Perception
- Mobilisation abilities
- Working and playing capacity
- Expression of sexuality
- Sleeping quality and memorising skills

Intervention can be put into three categories:

1   Physical care with a priority relating to alleviation of obvious risk factors and ability to carry out ADL

2   Emotional care

3   Social interaction with a consideration of what retained skills can be used positively in therapy.

Interventions have a two-pronged intent: to reduce unacceptable behaviour and to increase acceptable behaviour. Care planning also requires the taking of ideas from persons with dementia. They may be able to indicate their interests and the degree to which they can participate in the care plan.

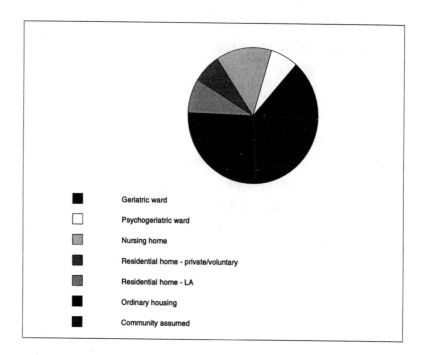

Figure 4.4: Place of residence of people 65+ years known to have memory problems and confusion

Source: Forth Valley Health Board (Dept of Public Health Medicine, 1994. Census of people aged 65+ with problems of memory and confusion, Gordon D, Scott S and Carter H

5
Dementia and dementia care — what are the alternatives?

" Henry sits alone outside the door to his room. He is pale and unkempt. There is a strong smell of urine in the air. Care staff walk past without acknowledging his presence. In the background there is the sound of laughter and enjoyment. However Henry sits in a world of isolation , loneliness and despair.

The care staff are asked for their perception of this man. They reply summarising their negative perceptions of a man who is someone's father, someone's husband and someone's friend. Henry continues to exist within his own world of solitude. Henry has dementia"

"Edith wanders from person to person. She is anxious and tearful. There is no one there to comfort her. She grabs at the nurses arm. The nurse pulls away and then walks away. A fellow resident shouts abuse at Edith. She wanders; she continues to wander aimlessly. Edith has dementia"

" Fred clings tightly to the hand of the social worker. The social worker and the nurse talk to each other. They collude to ensure that Fred remains within the unit. Fred, his eyes filled with fear and apprehension says nothing. His breathing is laboured and he waits for the social worker to make a move to get away. She breaks away; Fred reaches for her but she is gone. A grown man stands before a curious audience. Tears stream from his eyes. In despair he sits in a chair. He is left alone. Fred has dementia.

Introduction

Fred, Henry and Edith all suffer from varying degrees of dementia. However when I first met and assessed them they all presented with varying signs and symptoms of dementia. These three people have not however followed what many professional carers have come to see as the traditional model of dementia.

In fact far from seeing a decline in their mental state there has been a marked improvement in the level of their functioning.

In itself three examples prove very little. However there is a growing school of thought which suggests that there may be other ways of viewing dementia and, therefore, other ways of caring for people with dementia.

The aim of this part of the book is to ask the reader to consider alternative approaches to dementia care. To assist in this process the literature has been reviewed and some conclusions drawn from it.

Traditional approaches to dementia and dementia care

Kitwood (1988) describes the traditional view of dementia very much in terms of technical approaches. These views he concludes have guided many of the relatively fruitless attempts to find a cure for the illness.

Many of the assumptions underlying the care and treatment of the illness have not changed over the last thirty tears. Certainly nursing care has changed very little with a strong emphasis put upon physical care to meet the physical needs of the individual. Much of this care has been administered by demoralised staff working with limited resources. Overall this situation has represented an attitude to dementia care which has been far from innovative and enthusiastic. Indeed Larsson (1963) describes a bleak picture of the illness which he states is non-discriminating in who it affects — an illness with a prognosis of death within five to eight years. The course of the illness being progressive deterioration ranging from mild forgetfulness in the early stages to severe intellectual impairment and personality change in the final stages.

To those who care for the dementia sufferer and for those who are closest to them this traditional view gives no hope. It gives no hope for the sufferer and no hope for the carers.

'Michael's wife is visiting the nursing home. At the age of 77 she has to make the decision which will end a partnership of over 50 years. She recalls the roles which her husband has played and how much she loves him. She has cared for him for the past six months since he was diagnosed as suffering from dementia. She knows that the prognosis is poor. She knows that she can't care for him at home any longer. "What hope is there?" she asks'.

The illness is sometimes described as the *"death which leaves the body behind"*. This is a very negative view and if the sufferer is to receive the best treatment and support we must somehow consider dementia in a way which fosters hope and not despair. Once we can take steps to achieving this then we may start to see radical changes in the approach to dementia care.

Kitwood (1988) suggests that the approach to the illness from the caring professions has been to see the individual suffering from dementia in exactly the same way one would see a car which has broken down. That is to say a car mechanic may see a car which fails to start, identifies the cause, i.e. flat battery and then remedies it by some means or other. One could suggest that this technical approach has failed because although we have moved nearer to identifying the problem the cure remains illusive.

This technical approach has left nurses and nursing with a very minor role in the care of the dementia sufferer. Not minor however in terms of effort and the desire to help but certainly minor in terms of being able to influence the care which dementia sufferers and their families receive. It also generates feelings of guilt and helplessness within the families of sufferers at a time when they need to be at their strongest as more and more responsibility for the care of their relative is put upon them.

The technical or traditional view of dementia can and does affect the sufferers access to health and social care. This is because in some areas funding for the care of individuals is based very much on a medical diagnosis of mild, moderate or severe dementia.

This results in people with mild dementia receiving less financial and social support than those with severe dementia. In reality however, someone with severe dementia with lots of support networks may need less support than someone with mild dementia living alone in squalid conditions.

Formal and informal carers alike know only too well that the progressive deterioration of the individual cannot be totally explained in terms of purely technical processes. Our intuition tells us that something else is affecting the elderly person. For example, if this model was totally applicable to this client group we would not see what all carers see. That is the fact that one day the dementing individual can show all the signs of neurological and cognitive impairment and yet the next day they can be functioning at a much higher level .

I walk into the nursing home most mornings at around 9 o'clock. Fred shouts to me to attract my attention holding out his hand. He shakes with laughter as our banter amuses him. He presents me with a list of requests for the day. Cigarettes, batteries for his radio. The laughter is more intense as we continue our banter.

At this stage Henry can no longer resist making some sarcastic but very amusing comment and he then joins in the laughter.

Edith comes to me and we embrace. I compliment her on her appearance and she embraces me again. We walk hand in hand and we talk about whatever.

In the quiet part of the home Michael and his wife sit talking and having breakfast.

These are exactly the same clients described earlier in this chapter. However we can see that this snapshot of their behaviours and interactions has not deteriorated to the extent to which the traditional model would have suggested. Are we to assume that the brain cells which disappeared yesterday have returned today? This is most unlikely. Our experience as carers also tells us that changes in the person's functioning, temperament, mood and behaviour cannot be explained purely in terms of ongoing pathological changes.

As carers and as advocates we need to vigorously question views, beliefs, attitudes and practices. By doing this we have some hope of bringing about change in the care and treatment of individuals suffering from dementia.

Challenging the assumptions

I share the view that many of the assumptions of the technical approach to understanding dementia care need to be challenged. Indeed some of the basic assumptions were challenged over twenty years ago. Blessed, Tomlinson and Roth (1968) described the changes found in the brains of 50 patients at autopsy. The patients had shown signs of dementia prior to their death. Comparisons and measures were made to determine the nature of the changes associated with dementia in old age. On the basis of the changes found they were able to classify the brains into different diagnostic categories. They concluded in their major piece of research that the amount of neurological damage did not match with the level of signs and symptoms which the individual had displayed. Dementia, they concluded cannot be explained purely in technical terms and we have to therefore draw the conclusion that other factors come into play.

Several writers have written about "other factors" of dementia. Most of the work is unproven in the laboratory yet to carers it provides some explanation of what many observe and experience. Kitwood (1988) describes this as seeing dementia in personal terms. Seeing dementia in these terms means that we broaden our view of it from:

> Senile Dementia = Neurological Impairment.

to

> Senile Dementia = Neurological Impairment + Personality + Biography + Health State + Social Psychology

Kitwood (1993).

This equation, I believe, gives an exciting new opening for nurses and other carers alike in the care of the individual with dementia. It also provides a basis of hope for informal carers and the sufferer themselves. The traditional model has, as we have already discussed, tended to focus upon factors that have already happened or are as a result of pathological changes and are, therefore, very difficult to influence although they can be acknowledged.

The inclusion and acknowledgement of Social Psychology means that if indeed it does affect the individual and has a bearing upon the state of dementia itself, then we as carers can approach the situation with a greater feeling of being able to help provide a quality of life to the sufferer and their family.

Kitwood (1990) develops the personal framework further by stating that:

> Senile Dementia = Neurological Impairment + Malignant Social Psychology.

> Neurological Impairment attracts to itself a Malignant Social Psychology

> Malignant Social Psychology actually has a bearing on the level of Neurological Impairment and functioning of the individual.

It therefore follows that, if the level of malignant social psychology is reduced or the individual sufferer is protected from exposure to it, then the progression of the dementing process could be affected in a positive way.

It is worth spending a little time considering the nature of malignant social psychology.

Malignant Social Psychology

Kit wood's description of malignant social psychology and its effects is helping carers to re-examine their practices and is providing hope to the families of sufferers. It has helped us to be aware of our effects upon the individual sufferer. In other words although we go into the relationship to care for the person and we set up various policies and procedures to help us, we may in actual fact be harming the individual rather than helping.

Kitwood (1990) describes malignant social psychology as the processes which tend to depersonalise the individual. He describes ten aspects of malignant social psychology some of which we know that we have witnessed and unfortunately, in some cases, have been party to. He describes the following aspects of malignant social psychology and gives examples of it in practice I have given examples from my experience and it may be a useful exercise for any carer to reflect upon their practice and to identify areas of malignant social psychology which spring to mind.

I will draw upon the experiences of Fred, Henry, Edith and Michael to illustrate examples and I would ask the reader to refer to the accounts of them given at the beginning of this chapter.

Treachery: *Takes the form of trickery or deception.* Fred was told by the social worker that he was going for a ride in the car and after a visit to the nursing home he would return to the ward. Fred never returned to his ward.

Disempowerment: *Deskilling; Doing for.* Henry when admitted from home to the residential home was almost immediately put into incontinence pads. He was never given the opportunity to go to the toilet.

Infantalisation: *Inferences of the person having the characteristics and mentality of a child.* A well meaning carer attempts to comfort Michael's wife. "Don't worry" she says cheerfully, "they're all my babies, I'll look after him"

Intimidation: *Threats, impersonal approaches, abuse of power.* Edith refuses to take her medication and walks away from the carer administering the tablets."If you don't take these tablets I shall get you written up for an injection. The doctor will not be too pleased about that so you had better take them"

Labelling: *Diagnoses and self fulfilling prophecies.* Henry's cup of tea spills onto the floor. "He's done that on purpose you know. He's getting back at us for making him get out of bed so early"

Stigmatisation: *Exclusion, becoming an outcast.* Henry was the only person labelled with the diagnosis of dementia in the residential unit. Staff had come to some agreement that they would arrange the rota in a way that any individual member of staff would not have to 'deal' with him more than twice in a week.

Outpacing: *Caregivers continue at their normal pace.* Edith sits drinking a cup of tea. "Come with me" says the nurse. Edith continues to drink her tea with obvious enjoyment. The nurse takes the cup of tea and asks Edith to follow. Edith follows.

Invalidation: *Failure to have feeling and emotions understood or even acknowledged.* Edith is in a state of obvious distress. She approaches several members of staff but they prise themselves away from her or tell her to go and sit down.

Banishment: "Being sent to Coventry". Henry was not only stigmatised by the staff but by his fellow residents. He therefore spent most of the day sitting alone outside of his room.

Objectification: *Failure to be treated as a person.* The staff organising their work at the start of the morning shift, "I'll do the doubles and you do the singles. "The care worker agrees, "Oh yes and I'll do the respite"

On reflection, I'm sure we can all see examples of these in other care situations but I suggest that although they may happen in our care settings, they may not be as obvious. In many ways the examples of malignant social psychology are more subtle but they are there. What we have to be acutely aware of is that when the individual is exposed to malignant social psychology, they are being potentially damaged by it. It follows that we, as carers, have a duty and a responsibility to protect the individual sufferer from, or build their resistance to it's effects. Indeed, if the effects of these experiences are important then the carer who spends most of her time with the patient can make these experiences good or bad. However, perhaps the most important aspect of this alternative approach to dementia is that it actually gives carers a vital proactive role in the care of the dementia sufferer.

We can take steps to become aware of and reduce the level of malignant social psychology experienced by the individual. If we do this then if we consider the personal framework of dementia we can affect the persons quality of life and their well being.

The Human Experience of True Meeting

Perhaps the first step we should take is to explore how we see our selves and how we see those with dementia. Buber (1958) talks about the human experience of true meeting. Kitwood (1992) observes that we make a distinction between 'us' who are skilled and competent and 'them' (the sufferer) who are damaged and dependent. Whilst we continue to hold this view there can never be a true meeting of human experience. In other words we can never see the sufferer as equal. We can never come to terms with the fact that we may be damaged and damaging in some way (Mair 1989).

When we refer to 'we' in this context we must consider not those who provide direct care but perhaps also those who make policy and provide resources. As we start to critically analyse our beliefs and our practice we will start to acknowledge the individuals as equal partners in the caring relationship. In other words we acknowledge the personhood of the individual.

Personhood

Personhood is, essentially, a social concept (Kitwood 1993). It is consideration of the individual in relation to others (Gilleard 1989). It ascribes status to the individual which is worthy of respect (Kitwood and Bredin 1992). The recognition of the individual as a social being with status enables the nurse to use skills and relationships to maintain this social being. If we maintain or restore the social being then some of the neurological and cognitive functioning may be restored (Bell and Mcgregor 1991). The development of the culture of dementia where staff provide a highly stimulating environment can actually slow the processes down and stabilise individuals (Rovner *et al* 1990).

Already this is giving new hope and enthusiasm to carers who are themselves starting to question the therapeutic value of the traditional ward setting. Kitwood and Bredin (1992) suggest that, if we consider the personhood of the individual and reduce the effects of malignant social psychology, then dementia becomes far from being a hopeless case but a state in which even the most damaged of individuals can show signs of relative well being.

Wellbeing

Signs of wellbeing in individuals with dementia include the following (Kitwood and Bredin 1992):

Assertiveness

Initiation of social contact

Expression of a wide range of emotions

Affection

Warmth

Social sensitivity

Self respect

Humour

Creativity and self-expression

Helpfulness

Relaxation.

Think again of the examples I gave earlier in this work. Consider how the few individuals described moved from a state of obvious ill being to a state of social well being. No drugs, no therapies just respect, concern and love for those individuals.

Dementia care mapping

In order to do this a process called Dementia Care Mapping has been devised (Kitwood and Bredin 1992). It is a tool for measuring the quality of the individuals experience. Every five minutes their experience is categorised and allocated a letter. There are rules which govern the types of experience which take precedence over others. So far this seems little more than engagement studies which have been around for many years. The major difference is that every time the experience is categorised, it is given a care value. This care value ranges from

+5 to -5. We must see these care values as opposite ends of a scale. A score of +5 would be regarded as a highly therapeutic experience while a score of -5 would be seen as very damaging to the individual. For example, if we take the experience of eating and drinking. A score of +5 would involve 'eating a meal with some empowering experience, sociability or obvious enjoyment'. At the other end of the scale the same experience may score a -5 which would involve 'severely impaired independence, lack of desired sociability or complete dissatisfaction with food or drink'.

Recall also the fact that we are looking at the total global experience. We therefore make a note of any personal detractors which the individual may experience. A recent example of a mild personal detractor which I described earlier was a client having a nice cup of tea with fellow clients. (Care Value +5). A doctor then appears on the scene and says to the client, "come with me, I would like to ask you a few questions" The client says "let me just finish my drink" (signs of well-being, i.e. assertiveness). The doctor proceeds to take the cup from the patient and walks away with it saying "follow me". Here we have an example of some mild malignant social psychology, i.e. objectification and outpacing.

Each sufferer is 'mapped' over the six hour period. At the end of this we are able to present to the staff individual and group profiles. That is to say what were the most common experiences which clients within that area had, how long did they last for and what care values were attached to them. Once the data is analysed the most valuable part of this exercise is to give feedback to carers.

The important thing to remember is that it is up to the carers to draw conclusions from the data. They would be able to picture and 'experience' what the client was experiencing and the part they as a staff group played in it.

Once the conclusions have been drawn then the carers devise an action plan. Six months later the whole process can be undertaken again. Factors which have contributed to negative experiences which clients have been exposed to can be reduced.

Conclusions

The aim of this chapter was simply to ask the reader to reflect upon their own views, beliefs, attitudes and actions when caring for individuals who are suffering from dementia. The review of the literature suggests that there are alternative ways of considering dementia, ways which enhance the relative well being of the individual, ways which give hope to sufferers and carers alike.

The personal model or approach to dementia care provides a framework in which carers can deliver meaningful care and support. The model is one in which motivated carers and sufferers come together in equal partnership enabling the sufferer to remain a social being, to be respected and valued. Primarily, however, the alternative approaches described in the reviewed literature gives us all a sense of hope.

References

Bell J and Mcgregor I (1991). Living for the Moment, *Nurs Times*, **87(18)** 45–47

Blessed G, Tomlinson B E and Roth M (1968). The association between qualitative measures of dementia and of senile change in the cerebral grey matter of elderly subjects, *Br J Psych*, **114**, 797–811

Buber M (1958). *I and Thou*, Clarke, Edinburgh

Gelder M, Gath D and Mayou R (1991). *Oxford Textbook of Psychiatry*, Oxford Medical Publications

Gilleard C (1989). *Losing one's mind and losing one's place*, Address to the British Society of Gerontology

Jacques A (1988). *Understanding dementia*, Churchill Livingstone,

Kitwood.T (1993). Person and Process in Dementia, *Intl J Geriat Psych*, **8**, 541-545

Kitwood T (1990). The dialectics of dementia with particular reference to Alzheimer Disease, *Age Soc*, **10**, 177–196

Kitwood T (1988). The Technical, the Personal and the Framing of Dementia, *Soc Behav*, **3**, 161–179

Kitwood T and Bredin K (1992). Towards a Theory of Dementia Care, Personhood and Well-being, *Age Soc*, **12**, 269–287

Larson T (1963). Senile Dementia:A Clinical Socio Medical and Genetic Study, *Acta Psych Scand*, **167**, 1–259

Mair M (1989). *Between Psychology and Psychotherapy: Towards a Poetics of Experience*, Routledge, London

Roth M (1971). Classification and Aetiology in Mental disorders of Old Age, In: Kay and Walk (eds), *Recent Developments in Psychogeriatrics*, Headley Brothers, Ashford

Rovner B, Lucas Blanstein J, Folstein M F and Smith.S W (1990). Stability over one year in Patients Admitted to a Nursing Home Dementia Unit, *Intl J Geriat Psych*, **5**, 77–82

6
Cognitive losses and their management

Memory

A major problem for those dealing with dementia patients relates to the social interaction of communication. This involves cognition – *the mental processes by which knowledge is acquired, such as reasoning and perception.* Cognitive skills are controlled by the brain cortex and are often specifically affected by organic brain disease. The patient's disturbed thinking processes do not intermesh with the normal thinking responses of the carer, resulting in failure in two-way communication. Cognitive deficiencies refer to shortcomings in acquiring and manipulating knowledge. Affected individuals' display shortfalls in attention, imagery, memory, language, reasoning and perception. These elements encompass all aspects of human intelligence and loss of intellect invariably occurs with AD. The deficiency in cognitive skills varies markedly with the severity of the disease. In the early stages, some cognitive functions are more affected than others and some intellectual skills will decline more speedily than others.

Census

In a study by Forth Valley Health Board (1992), half the people identified as having memory problems were living in the community. Sixty-five percent of the reports on this sub-group came from GPs, district nurses and health visitors.

Memory defects in Alzheimer's disease

Memory impairment is often the first and most obvious indication of the onset of dementia. Different kinds of memory processes exist and there are variations in memory function with dementia.

Working memory

Primary or short-term memory is used for the temporary storage of information in everyday cognitive tasks and has very limited capacity, e.g looking up an unfamiliar telephone number and retaining it long enough to dial correctly. Information can be retained in working memory only for a matter of seconds unless it is actively refreshed by mentally repeating it over and over again.

In AD there is a deficiency in working memory, which is demonstrated in memory span tasks, e.g. the maximum number of digits a person can consistently hold in working memory — known as the digit span. Normal elderly people can hold around six or seven digits in working memory, whereas AD patients with mild to moderate impairment can only manage around five digits.

One way of testing the rate of forgetting from working memory is to give the patient a small amount of information to be retained, e.g. three letters. The patient is then prevented from refreshing the memory by being involved in a distractor task. He/she may be asked to remember the letters IBM and then to count backwards from 100 for ten seconds. After the ten seconds, the patient has to recall as many of the letters as possible. AD patients all show increased forgetting from working memory.

Long-term memory

A more permanent memory store, with a large capacity, is long-term memory, which can hold information for many years. It involves encoding, storage and retrieval and works like any filing system whereby new files are opened and references are catalogued and stored on a shelf or in a drawer until accessed again by the use of the catalogue reference. The cataloguing of the file is like the encoding process of long-term memory and AD patients have difficulty in coding information, especially new information

Although AD disturbance can create encoding deficiencies, long-term storage of the material, once in memory, is often little affected. Retrieval from memory stores takes place in response to a retrieval cue. The cue comes from something in the current personal status which provides a tip as to where the information is stored in long-term memory. AD patients have problems in retrieval, particularly where recollection is involved. **Recollection** is 'active retrieval' **where individuals have to work at finding answers** by generating their own personal retrieval cues, which is a common phenomenon in the ageing process.

Those affected by AD perform better in retrieval tasks if they are given some cues and, in general, unless specific retrieval cues are adequately provided for them, they will have difficulties in locating all the information held in their memories. Memory loss is often insidious and develops gradually with the occasional memory lapse and forgetting to perform a task. The distinction between dementia and reversible causes of memory impairment in the elderly may be unclear at this stage. Older people suffer from what has been called **benign senile forgetfulness**.

However, as the disease progresses, forgetfulness means that the AD sufferer is at risk from fire and other household hazards. Once the severe stage of the illness has been reached, patients forget where their relatives are and may even forget their own name. The therapeutic technique of **reminiscing** takes advantage of retained memory stores and is commonly used in the management of dementing patients to improve communication between patient and professional and family carer. Temporal and spacial disorientation associated with memory failure can result in behavioural problems.

Stages and development of memory impairment

Stage 1: **Mild memory impairment**
Mild memory lapses
Forgets errands
Fails to pass on messages

Stage 2: **Mild to moderate impairment**
Memory loss is more pronounced
Impairment significantly affects activities of daily living
May forget familiar people or friends
Disorientation in familiar surroundings
Confuses time of day or day of week

Stage 3: **Severe impairment**
Failure to recognise close relatives
Confabulation – creates untruths to fill memory gaps
Severe memory errors
Memory impairment creates safety problems
Memory loss is often considered the most prominent feature of dementia in the early stages and is a common problem which can have a devastating effect on the individual's ordinary life.
A characteristic feature of AD is the degree of **confabulation** associated with the memory loss.

Confabulation occurs when the person fabricates material instead of recalling information, but without being consciously aware of what he/she is doing. Confabulation can be

spontaneous, involving grandiose ideas which are false, or
provoked, which is a response to a particular memory cue that
has somehow become distorted.

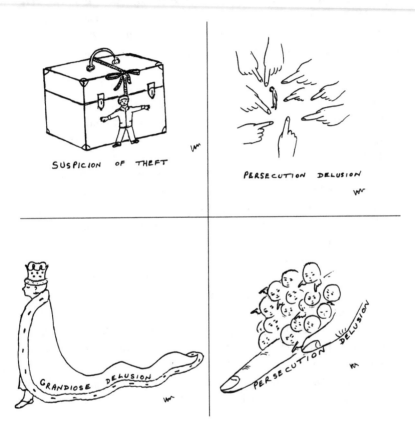

SUSPICION OF THEFT

PERSECUTION DELUSION

GRANDIOSE DELUSION

PERSECUTION DELUSION

In severe dementia, **delusions** occur. These are
disorders of thought content which are believed to relate to
memory failure. They may also be grandiose or persecutory in
nature, e.g. the patient may suspect that relatives or carers of
stealing from him/her.

Case history

A patient's severe behavioural disturbance and aggression against her nurses meant that a sedative injection was needed to calm her. She then made a formal complaint, charging the doctor of injecting her with the drugs in order to force her to leave her money to the hospital in her will.

Caution should be exercised before accepting such accusations as delusions however, as financial abuse of dementing patients does occur when carers are effectively embezzling funds or property from the affected person who is incapable of communicating the true state of affairs to the health professional. Sometimes failing memory leads the dementing patient to believe that the wife or husband is an intruder. The accuser's spouse finds this a difficult problem to cope with, when they are no longer recognised by their loved one and are seen as a stranger.

An understanding of these memory deficits will help the carer to accept some of the behavioural responses made by the patient. This information provision is often part of the attending nurse's role. Efforts can also be made to improve the memory and perhaps alter disturbing behaviour. The principal approach is memory management or memory retraining, which may be organised through a memory clinic (Wilson, 1987).

Rehabilitation approaches to memory management have to be pitched at a basic level of cognitive functioning. Often, the environment is structured to decrease memory requirements, teaching information is provided to the sufferer or efforts are made to change unacceptable behaviour. Simple strategies implemented by the community nurse or community psychiatric nurse can be of considerable benefit to patient and carer, and compensate for memory loss.

Nurses may be involved when carers approach them with complaints of behavioural problems. They can help to train the partners of dementia sufferers in simple behavioural procedures. For instance, carers can be taught to ignore their partner's suspicious and accusatory comments while reinforcing the patient's acceptable thoughts and behaviour through praise, touch and appropriate conversations. Spouses can be trained to ask questions, encouraging appropriate behaviour and then reinforce responses through touching, praising and smiling. Simple procedures, if structured appropriately, can change adverse behaviour significantly.

One approach in memory management or memory retraining (Wilson, 1987) is the use of systematic diary use or mnemonics.

Coping strategies

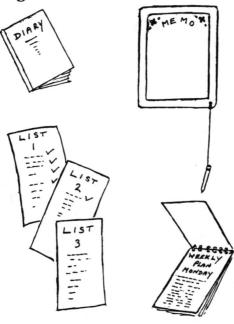

1	Mnemonics
2	The use of external records, such as diaries, lists, plans and diagrams
3	Verbal or auditory cues, such as alarms

4   Self-instruction — checking a task to see that it has
           been completed

These coping strategies can be of value, but if the patient denies
memory loss they may only provoke a hostile response. Several
other strategies are used.

Reality orientation has been used for many years and was
developed as a means of orientating a person to his/her
environment by means of continuous stimulation (procedures
which try to keep the confused in touch with personal facts and
their environment. Brook, 1975).

Twenty-four-hour reality orientation is designed as a means
of communicating with a dementia sufferer through their
waking hours:

a)   by restructuring the personal environment in the
           hope of improving orientation

b)   by communicating with the dementia sufferer using
           recurrent reminders

In everyday conversation, the person is reminded of their name,
where they are, current events of the day and the time of day.
The approach can be supplemented with changes in the
physical environment, such as installing clocks, calendars, signs
and pictures to improve orientation. For example, a pictorial
sign over the toilet door might encourage the use of the toilet.
Some demented people can perceive symbols better than
words, and both words and pictures may be of use, e.g. an early
morning approach by a nurse might be:

           'Time to get up now, sir, and get dressed'.

This could be altered to:

'*Good morning Mr Jones. I'm Nurse Smith. It's
your usual time to get up. It's eight o'clock.
Time to strip off your pyjamas and get into
your shirt and trousers. Breakfast is ready on
the table, over there*'.

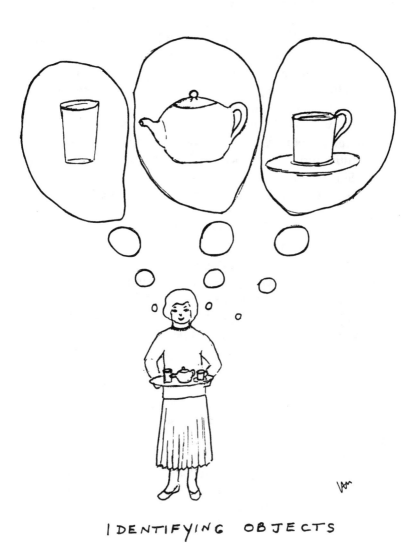

IDENTIFYING OBJECTS

Reality orientation

In reality orientation (RO), the patient is the focus of therapy and the technique encourages verbal orientation and functioning and improves cognition. Materials are used to focus attention and to improve orientation. RO does not work with those who are very confused, rambling and wandering. There is evidence that dementia sufferers can learn new information, although at a slower rate than normal (Morris, 1987), and can increase their level of knowledge through RO despite their illness. Using this strategy, patients have been shown to improve in ratings of self-care and socialisation.

RO was developed in the USA as an aide-centred activity programme for elderly patients. The procedure was thought to significantly improve functioning in dementing patients in the wards. Since then it has been subject to much criticism, but signposts around the home, depicting vital landmarks in words and pictures to assist orientation, are still commonly used, and RO is still considered to have a place in dementia care in the 1990s (Holden, 1990).

RO is now seen as an individualised 24-hour approach to developing a dementing person's strengths to meet his/her needs in relation to orientation and day-to-day memory. This individual focus identifies specific areas of orientation, such as keeping appointments and remembering specific events, and studies have shown significant cognitive and behavioural changes associated with 24-hour RO on an individual basis. The procedure should be seen as part of a range of options available in dementia care, but it has to be recognised that it is open to misuse when applied in a rigid and insensitive manner (Woods, 1994).

RO procedures demonstrate, however, that dementing patients do have learning potential and are still of practical use to nurses working in dementia care who should draw up management plans with specific goals of relevance to individual patients. Underpinning RO is the approach of the care-giver to the patient. The appropriate verbal and non-verbal communication does make a difference to the responses and behaviour dementia sufferers. Patients are known to show less difficult behaviour when care-givers remain calm and smiling (Crook, 1994). Orientation aids should be as much part of the care environment for dementing people as handrails are for those with physical disability.

Remembrance

The procedure involves looking back into the patient's past with his/her cooperation. People with dementia usually have much better recall of long-past life events than for recent events. Reminiscence allows people to recall the significance of their past and their status as a real person in the real world. It helps the carer to appreciate the patient's former standing in the community and his/her right to expect the same respect and standards of care in meeting the patient's needs as non dementia patients.

Not all memories are happy and care must be taken not to uncover tragic or unhappy events buried in the patient's past. The elderly have often lived through two world wars and will have experienced tragedy. It is preferable to avoid the recall of such unfortunate events.

Props such as old photographs, gramophone records, newspaper cuttings and memorabilia can be used to stimulate reminiscence. Sometimes the procedure will reveal parts of working memory still relatively untouched by the dementing process, e.g. singing, and the patient can be encouraged to explore this avenue of communication. The speech and singing centres are separated in the brain so that an aphasic patient may still be able to vocalise in song.

Case history

A male patient with multi-infarct dementia had been robbed of his speech and, on occasion, could be very depressed, frustrated and aggressive. Carers were struggling to maintain rapport with him. Attempts to improve communication using a conventional approach were unsuccessful and he began to withdraw into his own unhappy world. Unwillingly encouraged to join a sing-along one day, he suddenly found that he could sing and had an extensive repertoire of songs, learned in his past. This discovery completely altered his attitude and well-being. He regained a measure of self-respect because he was able to communicate with others and his new-found ability to participate in the sing-songs gave him intense pleasure. His aggression and depression disappeared and he established a good relationship with carers who found it humorous and fun to deal with him.

Memories help to put things into perspective and solve problems in the present. For the elderly and the dementing patients they can help to restore self-worth and esteem, buttressing up the present. Carers may come to appreciate the fact that the dementia sufferer is not just an empty shell but a real person entitled to good care and respect for his/her civil liberties.

Reminiscence uses past events and related objects to stimulate memory through recollection, whereas reality orientation stimulates the part of the mind that deals with time, place, persons and situations to which the dementing person may relate. A further consideration is **remotivation**, which is the testing and stimulation of the individual's intellect and cognitive characteristics through discussion, thought and deduction. Use of this 3R type of programme with patients can be effective for short-term mental stimulation of dementing elderly people (Koh *et al*, 1994).

Reminiscence therapy

Reminiscence therapy is used as an alternative approach to RO, often in a structured group in a day hospital or respite care setting, and many nurses use this technique very effectively. In this approach, there is an opportunity for dementia sufferers to review and reorganise events in their life. It encourages them to think and talk about past experiences through the use of memorabilia, pictures and slides. Popular among psychologists and occupational therapists, they believe it capitalises on preserving function. It helps patients to focus on positive past memories, avoiding potentially upsetting memories. Many carers find it an enjoyable activity with a personal focus on the patient. In the absence of other supporting health professionals, the nurse can instruct the family carer on some of the methods widely used in the therapy (Butler, 1963).

Reminiscence therapy has no clear focus but improves morale, and it can be used as an interaction activity. It is used to elicit memories and appears to improve orientation when combined with RO. Most patients find it enjoyable provided that they do not recall disturbing negative memories. It does not work with those who are very confused and rambling.

Validation therapy

The validation approach was developed as a more sensitive and empathetic procedure than RO (Feil, 1992). The approach does not insist upon participation in present reality and does not result in withdrawal of the patient. Validation has its strength in recognising that whatever words the patients use and whatever feelings they have are, in fact, true. Carers can, therefore respond to them without fear of promoting further confusion.

Words such as 'empathy' and 'understanding' are associated with validation and the procedure works on a feeling level. It should not be used in the disorientated AD patient. Validation has been defined as **an empathetic approach that affirms the personal reality of the demented elderly**. Empathy, it has been said, is the ability to walk in the shoes of the patient.

The validation method describes stages of progressive disorientation and offers specific techniques that can be used with each stage. It points care-givers, professional and familial, to a goal where there is acceptance that patients cannot be made better but can be helped along their path from whatever point they have reached.

Case history – Validation therapy

Diagnosed as Alzheimer's serveral years previously, Andrew, an old shepherd from the Highlands of Scotland, had a below-knee amputation and was readmitted with bad ulcers on his remaining leg which was incapable of bearing his weight. Carers found in-depth conversations with him very difficult, except on the subjects of sheep or cattle.

One afternoon at visiting time when the ward was full of visitors, I noticed that he was trying to rise from his chair. I went over and asked him where he was trying to go. Very loudly and angrily he replied, "How can you just stand there when there's a cow lying dead in front of you?".

As I tried to reason with him explaining that we were in a hospital ward, he just got angrier and his voice louder. Soon his wife came to visit. She asked how he was. He said he was very tired. She responded, "Oh, you've had a hard day tending the sheep then?" — **validation therapy**. *He quietened as she continued to speak to him of the animals that were once in his care*

A. Allison

The main goals of validation are:
- To restore of a feeling of self-worth in the patient
- To reduce stress
- To increase verbal and non-verbal communication
- To prevent inward withdrawal and to reduce the need for medication (Klerk and Rubin, 1994).

Validation therapy arose out of reactions to the insensitive use of RO. It involves listening with empathy to whatever dementia sufferers are trying to communicate about their current feelings (Feil, 1982). The aim is to validate the sufferer's conversation without correcting factual errors. The intent is to establish a two-way conversation between carer and sufferer. Claims for its value have been poorly evaluated. Both family and professional carers, including nurses, can employ these techniques in the community setting. While the behaviour of dementia sufferers can alter positively in response to these types of intervention, the changes in orientation and self-care can only be maintained with continuous input from the carers. The strategies have to be tailored to the individual, for each technique has the potential to make some sufferers distressed while being seen as a pleasant experience by others. A goal-planning approach for each individual sufferer has to be the objective.

Communication

Language — Poor quality speech, difficulty in finding the right words or the right names for objects and even **aphasia** can occur with dementia. As the disease progresses, speech can be lost entirely. Like normal individuals, those with dementia find greater difficulty in naming objects when the name appears less frequently in everyday language, but the importance of word frequency is more marked in those with dementia. Naming impairments are considered to be secondary to perceptual difficulties in identifying objects or pictures. Although vision may be unimpaired in AD, sufferers often have difficulty in recognising objects. The condition in which objects are seen but not recognised correctly is called **agnosia**. When agnosia is severe, faces of familiar people may not be recognised.

Visual spatial impairment — creates difficulties for dementia sufferers as they are unable to move about according to any plan. When demented patients become lost, they have difficulty in finding their way around their own house or in familiar surroundings. In general, comprehension i.e. understanding, of both spoken and written information is affected in dementia. There is some evidence that visual/perceptual deficits lead directly to behavioural problems (Henderson, 1989).

Guidelines for communicating with dementia sufferers

1   Be patient

2   Give the person time to respond

3   Be direct and consistent

4   Prompt with appropriate cues to encourage reminders and rejoinders

5   Use verbal and non-verbal approaches

6   Concentrate on feelings and try to get in touch with how the patient feels

7   Reassure and treat the patient with respect. Do not treat the patient as a child

8   Do not try to use reason or logic

9   Keep trying when there is obviously a failure in communication

10   It is better to withdraw if communication is impossible and try again later.

It is worth promoting good communication skills, for bad communication with the patient can lead to increased disorientation and aggression or, at best, frustration and apathy.

The following is a list of some of the barriers to good communications:

Communication Barriers in Dementing Patients

Environmental	— distractions like TV or the radio may attract attention
Sensory defects	— age-related defects in vision and hearing
Attitudes	— the patient may have no insight
Memory disability	— can affect concentration and the flow of conversation
Confusion	— the patient may be confused
Disorientation	— the patient may not know what day it is or where they are
Poor attention span	— inability to concentrate
Comfort status	— if the patient is physically uncomfortable, they may be preoccupied and unable to concentrate
Dysphasia	— the patient may not understand what is said (receptive) or be able to say what they want to say (expressive)

Communication barriers — carer with patient

Lack of background knowledge of the patient

Unhelpful attitudes	— patient is mad; cannot be helped; frightening; dangerous; should be in hospital; isn't my problem

Case history — communication impasse

Mr W, diagnosed with dementia four years previously, was registered blind and quite deaf. Born in London, he still had a strong cockney accent. He was admitted for a spell of respite care. One morning while giving out medicine with a colleague, we had a rather frustrating conversation. She approached him saying "I have your tablets here Mr W". "Fabric" he said. "Tablets" she said. "Hardwick, I think its somewhere near Manchester". I approached to 'help'. "Its your pills" I said. "She's asking me where Hardwick is" he said. I tried spelling out P.I.L.L.S. but he was still trying to remember where 'Hardwick' was. We left him for the time being. About an hour later as I was passing, Mr W called me over. He was holding an empty tissue box for discarding in the refuse disposal bucket and said "Could you ask them to put it in the bucket. Maybe you'd better spell it for them as they don't seem to understand."

A. Allison

Management of communication problems

Initially, there may only be difficulty in finding words or naming objects, in which case encourage the use of alternative ways of getting the message across, such as gestures or drawing pictures. Consider talking around the key word, asking for a description of the item that cannot be named. Use simple questions, such as 'Is it (a) or is it (b)?' and use cues and prompts. If the key word cannot be found, leave it and try again another time. Remember to remove external distractions and consider the use of object reminders. The following is a list of ideas for improving communication with the patient:

Improving communication with dementing patients

Verbal input

Volume	— speak loudly and clearly. Avoid shouting
Speed	— allow time for the patient to understand the content
Tone of voice	— speak in normal tones. Do not use baby talk
Appropriate choice of words	— Keep sentences short. Only proffer one piece of information at a time. Use experience to bridge past and present
Prompt	— Prompts can act as a reminder, e.g. identifies the person, the day of the week
Questions	— avoid open questions which can be difficult to interpret, e.g. what would you like to eat?

Non-verbal input

Eye contact	— face the person

Improving communication with dementing patients

Personal intrusion	— be aware of personal space. Stand close, but not too close, facing the person, within their line of vision
Facial expressions	— enhance communication; may be incongruous, e.g. inappropriate expressions for content of speech
Gestures	— use your own hands and arms to communicate; cosider the meaning of the patient's gestures
Physical contact	— a gentle touch helps alleviate anxiety. However, physical contact can sometimes be experienced as a threat
Environment	— Avoid distracting noises or interruptions

Common communication problems

Failure to understand instructions

- A professional carer should monitor the length or complexity of the instructions and reduce them to a level at which they may be understood. Instructions may be reinforced by non-verbal gestures.

Failure to sustain a conversation

- Keep the communication short and simple
- Keep reminding the patient of the topic of conversation and keep the topic specific

Failure to complete sentences

- Aid memory by repeating the beginning of the sentence
- Offer alternatives, if there is more than one possible ending

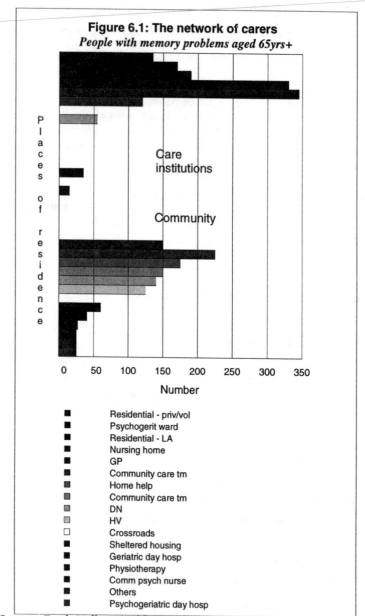

Figure 6.1: The network of carers
People with memory problems aged 65yrs+

Places of residence

- Residential - priv/vol
- Psychogerit ward
- Residential - LA
- Nursing home
- GP
- Community care tm
- Home help
- Community care tm
- DN
- HV
- Crossroads
- Sheltered housing
- Geriatric day hosp
- Physiotherapy
- Comm psych nurse
- Others
- Psychogeriatric day hosp

Source: Forth Valley Health Board (Dept of Public Health Medicine 1994)

* Use questions to remind the patient of the subject

Introduction of meaningless sentences
* Tell the patient that you have not understood
* Ask the patient to tell you again and cue into key words using non-verbal communication to help him/her understand
* If all of this fails, admit that the message has not been understood and try again later

Inappropriate topics
* Ignore the topic so as not to reinforce this behaviour
* Distract the patient on to another subject

Repetitive ideas and words
* Try to distract or divert the patient's attention
* Try to change the topic of conversation and stay away from topics that encourage this behaviour

The nurse does not only have to communicate with the patient; communication with the family carer is also important It may well be that carers have not chosen a caring role and refuse to accept it. If the onset of the role has been insidious, carers may not even recognise that they have become carers. It is important, however, that good information is fed to carers about the disease and the services and benefits available, and that they are encouraged to share their feelings. They should be encouraged towards contact with support groups.

The nurse also has to consider communication with other professional colleagues as communication frequently breaks down, to the disadvantage of everyone concerned. Every effort must be made to maintain good lines of communication between the members of the multidisciplinary team. This may be verbal or written. It is important that a good communication network is created and maintained. The network may be extensive, involving family carers, health professionals, social workers, voluntary agencies and lawyers (see diagram page 35).

7
Problem behaviour and its management

Few things are more stressful and emotionally exhausting for professional and familial carers than looking after people with persistent behavioural problems. It is important for nurses to recognise these pressures on the carer and to make every effort to alleviate them or ensure that there is adequate respite from the situation. In the long term, a day away or a proper holiday should be organised so that the carer may be absent from the scene for a while or, alternatively, a fortnight's residential respite care or temporary hospital admission may be arranged for the patient.

Managing disruptive behaviour

Disruptive behaviour can present in different ways. There may be:

- Overreaction
- Catastrophic reactions
- Wandering
- Sundown syndrome
- Aggression and violence
- Sexual overtones

Unfortunately, there are rarely quick-fix solutions to behavioural problems and the only practicable way is to take a step back and assess each coolly and and calmly. This is essentially a problem-solving exercise involving several steps:

1   Definition of the problem

2   Identification of possible causes

3   Decision-taking on appropriate action

4   Action and evaluation of response

It can be useful to differentiate between:

a)   Things which a person used to do for themselves but can no longer do

b)   Things which the person has started to do, perhaps for the first time. Often it is what the person cannot do that causes the problem. One has to keep in mind that the problem is not the dementing patients themselves, but what they do. The positive approach is to consider that difficult or anti-social behaviour is a management problem.

Potentially disruptive behaviour presentations

- Verbal rudeness, wild accusations and insistent demands
- Repetitive questions and actions — perseveration
- Screaming and shouting
- Emotional outbursts and overreactions
- Night-time restlessness
- Agitation
- Physical aggression
- Wandering
- Disinhibited toileting
- Uninhibited sexual behaviour

Each behavioural problem should be assessed separately and it is useful to ask:

1   What exactly happens?

2   When does it occur?

3   How long does it take?

4   Where does it occur?

Having described the behaviour, one should next try to understand the reasons for it. Factors contributing to challenging behaviour are loss of memory, inability to understand communications, the misinterpretation of conversations and the development of unrealistic beliefs or illusions.

Extreme emotional outbursts may result when the dementing person catches a glimpse of what is happening to him/her. It must be remembered that physical and sensory difficulties such as unresolved problems of failing eyesight and hearing can increase confusion or promote disturbed behaviour. These conditions have to be addressed and corrected. Old age and/or dementia are not unacceptable reasons for failure to provide spectacles or hearing aids when required.

Decisions on what to do revolve around:

1   Prevention

2   Toleration

3   Modification

These decisions are geared towards helping the individual to compensate for mental disabilities and RO can be useful in this respect. Independence has to be encouraged and individuals should be prompted to do small things for themselves. Provocation should be avoided. Toleration is not always possible, but in many circumstances potentially disruptive behaviour can be accepted as long as it does not cause harm. Disinhibited sexual behaviour falls into this category and, provided that the individual has some privacy, it may be acceptable.

It is not acceptable to physically restrain people who are exhibiting disruptive behaviour. This is an infringement of individual liberty. There are, invariably, other ways of dealing with the problem. Sometimes this may involve the use of medication to modify the behaviour.

It may be possible to alter the activating event or situation. There may be a trigger for the behaviour, and if this can be identified the behaviour may be avoided.

Another possibility is altering the consequences that follow the behaviour. Many behaviours are maintained by what happens in response to them. The behaviour may be attention-seeking; if the individual gains attention it becomes rewarding and the behaviour will become self-perpetuating.

Case history — Behavioural problems

Disruptive behaviour

Mr J was newly diagnosed as having dementia after a toxic confusion state was ruled out. He was very mobile, liked to be busy and watched and copied nurses. He began adjusting intravenous infusions, removing charts from the bottom of the beds and putting them under other mattresses. He gathered a pile of shoes from other patients' lockers to try on and, after watching the physiotherapist position chairs for transferring stroke patients to sit on them, repositioned them while she was moving the patient.

Staff found him odd jobs to do around the ward, i.e. helping to make beds, wash dishes etc, and his meddlesome, trying behaviour no longer presented as a problem.

A. Allison

Problem behaviours

Disruptive features occur with many dementing patients.

Agitation	— 85%
Wandering	— 60%
Depression	— 60%
Screaming	— 25%
Violence	— 20%

Rapp M S, 1992

Agitation and restlessness

Agitation has been defined as inappropriate verbal local or motor activity that is not explained by the individual's apparent needs or current state of confusion. Three agitation syndromes have been described:

1   Physical aggression

2   Verbal agitation

3   Disruptive motor function without vocal involvement or physical agression

It may occur in as many as 85% of demented patients.

Disruptive vocal behaviour

Disruptive vocal behaviour comprises screaming, moaning and repetitive calling. **Perseveration** is the constant repetition of a word or phrase; this can be very irritating and even repeated gestures may be annoying. It is important for the carer to respond not to the perseveration itself, but to lack of it. If possible, it is better to interrupt before it becomes established. Repeated 'calling out' can be reduced by increased personal contact and systematic observation to identify patterns, times and situations when the behaviour occurs. This may often uncover its meaning. It may be that the patient is seeking toileting or other comfort needs. If the repetitive conduct, shouting and 'calling out' is attention-seeking, the inappropriate behaviour should be ignored and the appropriate behaviour rewarded in an effort to halt the disruptive response. Screaming may be a feature in 25% of dementing patients.

Overreaction

Dementing patients often react to very minor criticisms or a trivial setback with a gross emotional overreaction. They respond with screaming, shouting or unreasonable accusations. This tendency to overreact may cause them to become suddenly very agitated or they may refuse to move. This is known as a **catastrophic reaction** and refers to an exaggerated response which is quite inappropriate to the remark or event that is the trigger.

Catastrophic reactions may appear as emotional lability, inconsolable crying, anger, increasing restlessness or pacing, or aggressive or sudden stubbornness. It is thought that these reactions occur most often in response to overwhelming environmental stimulation, such as when dementing patients are asked too many questions at once, when there are too many strange people about or when they have been scolded or confronted. They can, however, occur when sufferers fail to succeed at a simple task.

It is important to remember that the behaviour is secondary to brain damage and not under personal control. The patient may well be quite frightened and need reassurance. The situation is best dealt with by remaining calm, offering reassurance and endeavouring to distract attention. Reprimanding or punishing the sufferer is inappropriate. There is often a few minutes warning before an outburst when there may be increasing agitation, and the professional carer should be able to prevent the reaction escalating through immediate reassurance or distraction. The nurse involved should not feel that the reaction is directed at him/her personally. Slow, reasonable conversation with a limited series of questions and simple tasks without too great an expectation of the patient may prevent these reactions.

Anger and hostility

Physical violence may be exhibited in 20% of dementing people. This may present as yelling, cursing or belligerence, and should be seen, if possible, as a normal reaction to the losses imposed on the individual by the disease. Causes may be multiple, as there may be physiological, social or mental reasons for the behaviour, which may be related to the premorbid personality or even to a lack of awareness of the patient's physical limitations by the carer. Try to understand the reasons behind the behaviour and try to modify it. It can be difficult for those caring for dementing patients to appreciate the devastating loss of self and self-esteem engendered by this disease. Empathetic listening helps.

A calm and consistent routine, without excess stimulation, and the application of reality orientation may help to alter excessive behavioural responses. It is important to reinforce the remaining capabilities of the dementing patient and not just to focus on his/her disabilities.

Case history — Empathetic concurrence

Mr H was diagnosed as suffering from dementia five years previously. The junior doctor did an MMSE on him. When asked how old he was he answered 77. His real age was 87 but he got his date of birth correct. The doctor tried to show him that the date he had given as his date of birth subtracted from that day's date proved that he was in fact 87 years of age. Mr H went quiet and became visibly upset. Once the doctor left, he approached in some agitation with a piece of paper with the sums on it.

"That doctor is trying to say I'm 87. I would know if I was 87, but I'm only 77" he shouted angrily. I too tried to show him that by subtracting his date of birth from the year's date, the answer was 87. He took the paper and studied it, then asked another nurse to look at it. His anger and agitation increased and he was clearly unhappy. I went over to him and looked at the paper. "I'm sorry Mr H, I've made a mistake; you are only 77; I was wrong". Mr H reverted to his usual happy self once more. At the price of a little white lie, he became a contented patient again.

A. Allison

Although the mental distress experienced may be related to the disease and the patient's awareness of loss of control over the activities of daily living, it may also result from the attitudes and behaviour of carers who may be restraining or babying the patient, treating him/her disrespectfully, or even using physical abuse. Physical symptoms also have to be considered. Problems that are common in old people are just as common in the elderly with dementia. They too may have problems with constipation or bladder control, and may be lonely and depressed. The distress caused to patients and carers by physical problems can often be markedly reduced by advice and simple training from the community nurse. For example, constipation due to poor diet and immobility can be improved with medication and dietary supplements. Regular bladder emptying is recommended. Underlying disease, e.g. anaemia, chest and urinary infection should be treated and its presence promptly drawn to the attention of the doctor.

The nursing process for care interventions

- Assess
- Plan
- Implement
- Evaluate

Assessment focuses on the circumstances of the aggressive acts. Questions that should be asked include:
- What is happening?
- When does it occur?
- At Whom is it directed?
- What is the response of other people?

Management involves trying to alter the circumstances of a response by other people so as to make the aggression less likely or its impact less problematic. However, there are times when the agitation will escalate and recourse to medication may be necessary. The exclusion of possible toxic physical causes of confusional states must be kept in mind.

Greene (1979) showed that unstable mood embodying aggression, anger and accusation was patient behaviour that carers found difficult to cope with. It had a more discouraging effect on them than failures in their charges' functional ability. Nurses felt embarrassed, angry and frustrated and often became depressed and felt that their own health was deteriorating.

Psychological treatment is tailored to the specific behaviour problem, whereas **drug treatment** is rarely specific and the same medication is likely to be recommended for wandering, aggression or sleep disturbance. Commonly used drugs are chlorpromazine, thioridazine and haloperidol. They reduce overall activity which can help to make the behaviour or disturbance less of a problem. They all have side-effects, some which are quite marked, and they are not specific cures for particular problems.

These drugs are major tranquillisers and in some cases can add to the problems caused by dementia if they are given without close monitoring, for a prolonged period and in too high a dosage. Minor tranquillisers, such as diazepam and nitrazepam, are also used. These drugs essentially work by making the patient drowsy. A major problem of all drug therapy is that it may exacerbate confusion and can itself cause confusion through side-effects.

Overall management includes simple procedures with psychological treatment and drug medication focusing on the individual. Aggressive outbursts, wandering, sleep disturbance and perseveration are major sources of distress to both carer and patient. They can also be very disturbing for the attending nurse and it should be accepted that therapy is often a compromise between over-sedation and unacceptable social behaviour.

Early intervention before the situation reaches crisis point is always the best approach, but this is only effective if the situation is consistently and sensitively monitored. The district nurse, in her traditional role, and the community psychiatric nurse (CPN) in a newer role, with their regular domiciliary visits are particularly suited for this task. Active intervention with the intention of promoting change has to be monitored however, and the need for regular reassessment of the health status and needs of the patient should be borne in mind. The selective use of affective touch — the nurse touching the patient in empathy at a time unrelated to a physical care task — in a gentle reassuring manner can be therapeutic (Seaman, 1982). It can improve communication with or calm the confused or agitated patient. Burnside (1981) has shown that by increasing use of nurse/patient touch there is an increase in appropriate verbal communication and eye contact in elderly people with chronic brain disease.

Wandering

Wandering is common with this type of patient, affecting 60%. As dementia develops, a common feature is the liability of the sufferer to wander away from home or from where he/she is expected to be. A failing memory and declining communication skills may make it impossible for carers to discover why the patient has wandered off. Since sufferers cannot be imprisoned in their own home, one has to accept a degree of risk in their care and allow them a certain degree of personal liberty. However, fear of wandering and risk to the wanderer make this option a major social concern for family carers. The onset of wandering often brings calls for the nurse or doctor to seek institutional care.

The word 'wander' means ramble or move with no definite objective. In fact, in dementing wanderers, there are often underlying reasons for their wandering, although they may not be able to work them out. A management plan should initiate a search for these reasons. Some people wander because they feel uncertain and disorientated. Much of this is due to loss of short-term memory and the individual is unable to remember where he/she has gone or why. Is it wandering or is she/he just walking about (McShane, 1994)?

It can, however, be a means of using up excess energy. Those who have been used to walking long distances when younger may just be continuing the habit. It may be a means of expressing boredom. As dementia progresses, people find it harder to concentrate for any length of time on previously interesting activities and any activity becomes more difficult. Any source of agitation may cause people to pace up and down or wander off for no apparent reason. There may be perceptual problems and patients may fail to recognise their own home. A common cause of wandering, which is frequently overlooked, is that patients may be experiencing pain or discomfort but are unable to communicate their needs. They may be constipated, have toilet access problems or be suffering from more generalised pain. People sometimes leave the security of their own home because they are mistaken about the time, believing that they ought to be carrying out a task elsewhere. They may even be seeking companions who are now dead, or long departed from the scene.

Nocturnal wandering

As people with dementia often suffer from disturbed sleep, they awaken in the early hours and may become disorientated and liable to wander. Professor Mary Marshall from the Dementia Services Development Unit, Stirling University, believes that wandering is a myth and that one should concentrate on the fact that demented people walk and that there are reasons why people walk, which should be sought (Marshall, 1993).

Possible reasons for wandering (Allan, 1994)

1   Searching: Looking for a deceased spouse or their own home

2   Boredom: No activities to keep them occupied

3   Loneliness: Looking for familiar companionship

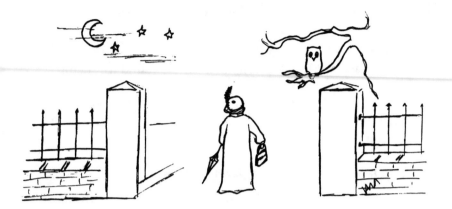

NOCTURNAL WANDERING

4 Separation: Anxiety about some other person

5 Forgetfulness: Forgetting the correct time to go shopping or visiting

6 Physical discomfort

7 Disorientation: This is particularly likely if they are moved to strange surroundings, e.g. when moving between sibling homes, day centres or respite care environments

8 Attention-seeking

Management involves seeking the the cause and several questions should be asked:

- What is being looked for and is it available in the home? If so, can it be shown to the patient or is there a suitable alternative?

- Where is the individual trying to go and is it a safe place for them to visit alone? Can they visit on their own with practice or can they go there with someone else?

- Who are they looking for? Is it someone who is available? Is it someone that can be found for them?

Patients who wander should be provided with an identification bracelet which can be worn at all times. These are available from an organisation called MEDIC ALERT.

Case history — Directive intervention

Mr C cared for by his wife in a big house with large grounds. *An ex cabinet-maker, he suffered from a cerebrovascular accident and was left with some limb weakness and swallowing problems. On his first day in hospital intravenous infusion was attempted. After the IV line was removed by him six times, it was decided to let him eat a modified diet and thickened fluids. This was successful.*

A very stocky powerful man, he wanted to go home and physically lifted a nurse from the exit door when she tried to prevent his exit. I told him the door was jammed Being a cabinet-maker he wanted to fix it. I led him to a cupboard door and left him to potter about happily. When he became over-demanding, I also asked him to check the locker doors and drawers. This controlled his restlessness and kept him happily occupied for a time.

A. Allison

There are now a number of electronic aids available for monitoring a patient's wandering. A small tag is secured about the patient's person and an electronic exit marker is placed on any doorway by which the patient might attempt to leave the residence. If the marker is passed, the tag completes an electronic loop which activates an alarm system similar to that which operates in shops. It does away with constant surveillance but many people feel that tagging is an infringement of personal dignity. The use of restraining chairs, with clip-on tables and other physical restraints that prevent the confused getting up and wandering freely about the room, must be condemned. They are a denial of personal liberty and dignity. If the cause of the wandering cannot be discovered or the behaviour altered, the use of a minor tranquilliser can occasionally help. Thioridazine 25 mg at night or 10 mg during the day at the time when the wandering usually occurs can be useful. A nocturnal sedative such as temazepam may improve sleep and diminish wandering and the occasional use of a minor tranquilliser such as diazepam can be useful.

Chemical restraints using drugs are sometimes necessary, but their use should be minimal and, ideally, short-term as they can cause daytime sedation and drowsiness leading to confused states. A review of current medication is necessary when assessing agitated behaviour.

Facts to remember

- Mental restlessness, linked with physical restlessness, may be related to feeling lost and not belonging
- Lack of exercise and boredom increase the risk of wandering
- Look for patterns and the time of day that triggers the wandering, and try to understand what is going on in the patient's mind
- Dementing people have a right to explore their environment and their freedom to do so should not be curtailed
- Physical and chemical restraints should be used only rarely

Questions to be considered

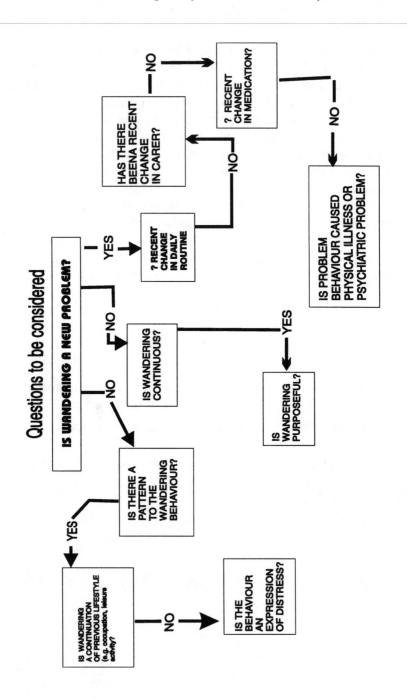

Withdrawal

The dementia itself may not necessarily be the cause of withdrawn behaviour. Depressed mood is a very common cause of 'withdrawal' and is treatable with medication.

Case history

Mrs Jones asked her GP for help with her husband, a former outdoor enthusiast. He had given up driving after a few minor mishaps which were his fault. He now refused to go out or even visit or see friends at home.

He had lost confidence in himself, was full of self doubts and was frustrated at loss of former skills and freedom. He had a poor memory and occasional flashes of ill-temper which he could not control in public. Sleeping through the night was also a problem as he only slept for short periods.

In assessment, he was physically sound but had signs of early dementia. He also scored high on the Hamilton Rating Scale for Depression. He responded to antidepressant therapy and later cognitive therapy from the clinical psychologist. He was encouraged to discuss his doubts about his mental state and became less withdrawn and more at ease with himself and others once his violent outbursts ceased. His sleep pattern also improved and so did the health of his wife as she no longer faced the day half asleep after disturbed nights.

Dealing with withdrawn behaviour

Depression can occur in as many as 60% of dementia patients and may cause a retreat into isolation and withdrawal. There are a number of reasons why people with dementia may seem withdrawn. These include fear of failure in carrying out normal activities of daily living, loss of self-esteem, silent protest, lack of control, apathy and reclusiveness. Withdrawal is not uncommon in dementing patients and is made worse by the decline in communication skills.

Careful assessment of withdrawn behaviour can indicate possibilities for intervention. Recognition that loss of old skills, freedoms, activities and roles can lead to feelings of helplessness and demoralisation can help those undertaking intervention. Withdrawal is often a sign of the patient's distress.

Management plan

1   Assess physical condition and medication

2   Make a behaviour assessment

3   Undertake psychological assessment of thoughts and attitudes

4   Assess the interpersonal situation with members of the family

5   Exclude drug medication as a cause

An interactive contact method of managing the patient uses bodily contact and communication skills to gain attention or show that someone is interested and values interaction.

Insomnia and altered sleep patterns

A common problem with dementing patients, more marked in the middle and late stages of the disease, is disturbance of the sleep/wake cycle. Typically, affected people have little difficulty in falling asleep but awaken during the night. They then get up, possibly for toilet reasons, and pace about, wander, attempt to leave the home, become disorientated and are unwilling to return to bed.

This can be particularly stressful for family carers who suffer disturbed nights which undermine their own health. They are also seriously concerned that the patient may wander out of the home late at night or in the early hours of the morning, inadequately dressed. Interference with sleep is commonly seen in depression, although often the disturbed sleep pattern consists of an inability to fall asleep or early morning wakening. Management should include a search for specific reasons for the nocturnal wakening with a review of medications, pain control, need for the toilet, lack of daytime exercise or excessive day-time napping.

Useful management techniques include:

- A routine of daytime activities, exercise and rest
- Anticipation of toilet needs by provision of bedside commodes or urinals
- A lighted route to the toilet or some kind of night light left on
- Avoidance of beverages containing caffeine and heavy meals late in the evening
- Establishing consistent bedtime rituals and discouraging excessive daytime napping
- Treatment of depression or pain
- A review of medications to rule out the possibility of adverse side-effects

Sundown syndrome

This is the term given to confusion occurring in the late afternoon or early evening. It may be caused by drug medication; monitoring the drugs and reducing the dosage may prevent the disturbance. Another possible cause is dehydration and adequate fluid intake in the afternoon may reduce the occurrence. It is not delirium (Bliwise, 1994) nor is it unique to dementing patients as it occurs in other brain disease.

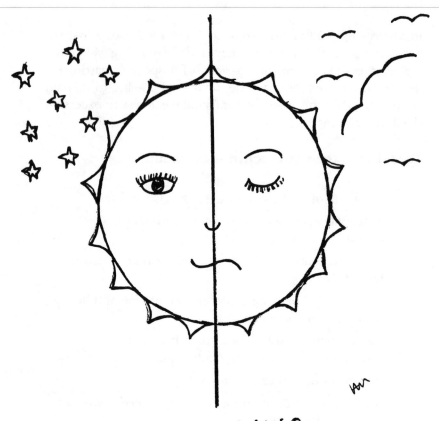

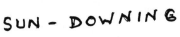

SUN - DOWNING

8
Sexuality and dementia

Sexual problems and dementia

The nurse may meet management problems or feel ill at ease or unable to cope when faced with overt and inappropriate sexual acts or sexual advances by the patient. He/she may also be the recipient of confidences from the caring spouse concerning worries, fear and guilt in the couple's sexual relationship. The sexuality of old people has received little investigation and, until recently, has been regarded as inappropriate or immoral. There is now an appreciation that expression of sexuality and sexual activity does not stop at 70 years of age, although little is known about how much, how often and what type of heterosexual or homosexual behaviour is enjoyed by older couples.

Sexual activity in the old is not exceptional and tends to be a continuation of lifelong patterns. It is certainly more important than was previously acknowledged, although people may be reluctant to talk about their sexual feelings. Equally, there is a reluctance on the part of health professionals to treat or refer elderly people with sexual dysfunction. It is known that men who continue to make love to their demented wives generally remain more effective carers (Kellit, 1989). Sexual activity of any kind has to be seen as a mutual expression of love and when problems arise, they should be considered and a management plan put in place (see Framework for Action)

The attending nurse should ask:
- Is there a problem?
- For whom?
- What action is appropriate?

- Once instigated, is it of use?

The problem may be a simple one.

Case history

A patient, a retired headmaster, was wakening in the early hours, sitting on the edge of the bed and masturbating. He would, thereafter, get up and urinate in the corner, to his wife's great distress. This patient's main problem was an urge to pass water and he was disorientated and deluded. He was unaware of his actions during the night. A mild sedative in the evening helped him to sleep through the night and the problem was resolved.

A common problem is 'self-exposure' and masturbation in public which may be associated with wandering. If the cause of the wandering is addressed, masturbation in public may cease. Some dementing patients have damage to the frontal lobes of the brain which can lead to disinhibition. The individual may have kept homosexual tendencies secret for many years and the sexual advances made by the patient may be a continuation of past repressed behaviour. Equally, disinhibition of the frontal lobes may result in the patient displaying inappropriate sexual behaviour and making offensive remarks. It may also be that, with the short-term memory disturbed and only long-term memory surviving, memories will include sexual abuse as a child which has been repressed and is only revealed with the onset of dementia. Some behaviour, which appears to be sexual, may be an expression of toilet needs, e.g. a woman lifts up her skirts and a man fumbles at his trouser buttons.

Discussing the patient's sexual behaviour with a spouse may be seen, indirectly, as discussing that person's own sexual feelings and behaviour. This may create a problem for the spouse. Older carers are reluctant to report sexual difficulties and even more reluctant to seek help. Of 242 referrals to a marriage and sex guidance council clinic in Sheffield, only three were over 70 years of age (Archibald, 1994).

Problems between spouse and the demented patient

Women may worry about rejecting advances from their husbands in case they wound their pride. Excessive sexual demands may be made of the spouses, who may already be deprived of proper sleep as a result of disinhibition. The demented patient may also exhibit inappropriate sexual behaviour in public. Loss of libido in the dementing patient early in the disease process may also be a cause for concern. Equally, the caring partner may feel guilty after having found another partner to satisfy his/her sexual needs.

One model of management worth considering when the nurse is approached is the Plissit Model (Annon, 1976). It offers four levels of sexual counselling and the nurse can use the level of intervention with which he/she feels most comfortable.

1   Giving permission. The nurse indicates to the carer that he/she is willing to discuss sexual thoughts and feelings

2   Offering limited information. It is useful to reassure a carer that the partner's aberrant sexual behaviour is the consequence of the illness and not a reflection on the couple's relationship. It has to be acknowledged that both partners may still have sexual needs and feelings. If frequent sexual demands are made due to loss of short-term memory, reminders that activity has just taken place may help. If the carer feels that he/she cannot respond to repeated sexual requests, the demands may be met by responses offering physical closeness and reassurance.

3   Involvement of others in the health care team. Not all nurses will feel comfortable offering sexual counselling and recourse can be made to other members of the health care team. Many GPs have counselling expertise and health visitors are

developing new skills in this area. Many places have a psychosexual referral service or the psycho-geriatrician can be approached for assistance.

Sexuality is one aspect of normal life and part of normal behaviour and problems relating to it should be dealt with in a similar fashion to other behavioural problems. Where there is loss of libido, carers may need to find a way of developing other means of sexual gratification. If this loss is the result of medication, the drug regimen should be reviewed. Alternative means of sexual expression might be encouraged, such as activities that do not involve intercourse, e.g. mutual manual stimulation, masturbation, massage, holding and hugging.

Many drugs e.g. beta blockers, do suppress sexual drive, which may already be waning in the elderly. A close review of the drug regimen should be carried out. Management alternatives to the use of medication to control or stop obtrusive sexual behaviour should be fully explored before recourse to drug treatment.

Case history — Sexual provocation

Mr L was in the early stage of dementia. He exhibited lots of denial and was very plausible. He liked to be wheeled to the toilet rather than use a urinal or commode by his bed. He told me the reason was because he always continue to get a cuddle from the nurse who brought him down. He also habitually made other sexually suggestive comments to the female staff. This made the staff uncomfortable and most of them avoided taking him to the toilet and spent as little time as possible with him. Perhaps if they had offered a therapeutic touch or a cuddle during normal nursing procedures in the ward, he might have been helped to cope with his sexual needs more appropriately.

Adverse features which may affect sexuality

- Illness
- Diabetes
- Incontinence
- Angina
- Stroke and Parkinson's disease
- Arthritis
- Gynaecological problems
- Psychological disturbance
- Anger
- Depression
- Guilt

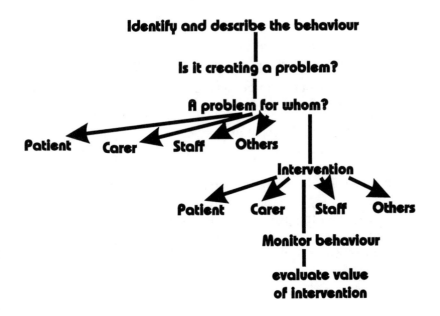

Framework for Action

Identify and describe the behaviour

Is it creating a problem?

A problem for whom?

Patient   Carer   Staff   Others

Intervention

Patient   Carer   Staff   Others

Monitor behaviour

evaluate value
of intervention

Incontinence of urine and/or faeces

The desire to pass urine may cause men to expose their genitals in public, behaviour likely to be regarded as indecency but is in a result of disinhibition. Removal of wet or soiled clothing in inappropriate places may also be misinterpreted. Dealing with the incontinence may prevent the embarrassing behaviour. Incontinence of urine and especially of faeces is often the final indignity for the carer trying to cope with a dementing patient at home. Fortunately, urinary incontinence is far more common than faecal incontinence, and usually occurs in the later stages of the disease.Urinary incontinence is one of the principal reasons for the involvement of the community nurse in a household where there is a dementing patient.

Management is the same as for other any incontinent person with an initial search for specific clinical causes. If these cannot be remedied, there must be a discussion with the carer as to the most appropriate ways of managing the problem.

Assessment should include the following questions:
- How long has it lasted?
- How often is the person wet or soiled?
- Do they simply forget where the toilet is?
- Do they need encouragement or frequent reminders?
- Is there a functional or physical cause of the problem, e.g. an infection?

The nurse should always remember that, while this may be a source of annoyance for the carer, it can be embarrassing and humiliating for the patient. Regular toileting at set intervals may help in many cases. Observation for signs of fidgeting, pulling at the clothes or wandering may alert the carer to the need for toileting.

Case history

A retired cleric repeatedly fumbled with his trouser fly buttons and exposed himself while at home. This only became a problem when he did so in front of some teenage girls. He had been exhibiting urinary frequency for some time which required many visits to the toilet. The urine was checked at the laboratory, an E. Coli infection demonstrated and treated. This cured the frequency and the acts of exposure ceased.

Clothes should be easy to remove or unfasten. The use of tracksuit trousers, full skirts and Velcro fastenings are advantageous. The occupational therapist can be approached to advise on adequate toilet and bathroom aids, and reality orientation can be used to signpost the way to the toilet. At night, a nightlight left on may facilitate normal toileting and the use of commodes and bedpans may be helpful.

If these measures fail, the usual continence aids should be supplied together with the provision of a linen-laundering service. The incontinent patient should have a midstream specimen of urine tested by the laboratory for bacteriology and a urine check for sugar should be carried out exclude diabetes. The possibility of prostatic problems should also be explored by the GP and hypertrophic prostatism excluded as a possible cause. 'Conveen' sheaths and in-dwelling catheters are poorly tolerated by dementing patients and recourse to continence pads may be necessary.

9
Caring for the carer

About 80% of dementia sufferers are thought to be living within the community, and the Community Care Act 1990 which was implemented in 1991, makes it likely that even more people with dementia will continue to live at home in the future. There are financial advantages to the health and social services in keeping such patients in the community. It has been noted by the Director of the Alzheimer's Disease Society, Dr Harry Cayton, that an hour of support care a week for a carer of a person with Alzheimer's disease (AD) in its early stages may be sufficient to keep that person out of hospital for a very long time. If there is no care, however, a state of crisis management persists.

A survey of 1303 carers conducted by the Alzheimer's Disease Society (1993) revealed that 50 % of carers spend more than 80 hours per week caring for a relative or friend with the disease. Ninety-seven per cent of respondents were experiencing emotional problems, stress, tiredness, depression or loneliness. Forty-one per cent of carers had drawn on private savings, taken out a loan or sold property in order to meet the cost of caring.

It is now the responsibility of local authorities in collaboration with medical, nursing and other interests to assess individual needs, to design care arrangements and to secure their delivery within financial budgets. They meet this obligation through social work departments, which usually appoint a case manager to assess individual needs and consider the difficulties; the assessment is done by social workers.

Considerable pressure is exerted on the physical and emotional reserves of carers who may have to cope for up to a decade with their debilitated spouse or sibling. The need for constant care restricts the carer's own lifestyle and quality of life. Carers become mentally exhausted and can easily become isolated from society and trapped in what has been called the 'ongoing bereavement' of involvement with a dear one suffering from AD.

Case history

Tommy had been a professional 'in the City'. Reluctant to leave this hub of activity, he was forced into early retirement to care for an ailing wife. With no family or close relatives, he found himself in sole charge of his 76 year-old wife who had suffered from Parkinson's disease for fifteen years.

She had become almost a total invalid and Tommy fed and cared for her throughout their waking day. Sadly, she also showed symptoms of dementia. Her memory, once sharp, became faulty. Once calm and patient, she became noisy and verbally abusive. She would sit and repeat his or her name for half-an-hour unless distracted. Delusions began to creep into her thinking and she would talk to her long-dead father who she said was sitting beside her. Tommy was remarkably tolerant and patient with her as her home-care came to dominate his life.

He ultimately only went out to shop and had no breaks or holidays. Latterly, she began to forget who he was, identifying him as a stranger who she roundly berated for getting into bed with her. Even when she became occasionally physically abusive he struggled to support her needs. Gradually, she began to turn night into day and he lost sleep and weight because of the continual demands. The last straw was the onset of incontinence which was also associated with her undressing, irrespective of environment.

Efforts to provide home-help and nursing support to maintain her in the community failed and she was admitted, initially for assessment and then placed in a long-stay ward. Tommy's own health had been undermined in his battle to provide her with care and he died long before his wife. Despite his devoted care, he felt guilty at allowing her to be institutionalised, grieved for the loss of his loved one and, although he went to see her almost daily, he became very depressed prior to his death.

Emotional problems arising in carers

Anger and **aggression** commonly occur when the carer feels fatigued and frustrated, and these can be signs that the carer is reaching the end of his/her tether and requires further help.

Role reversal may be a problem for children who suddenly find themselves with dependent parents, or for a very dependent wife or a non-domesticated husband who has to take up the burden of running the house and caring.

Guilt may develop in carers for a number of reasons, such as:
- Losing their temper with the patient
- Not wishing to carry the burden of responsibility
- Absenting themselves from care
- Placing the patient in respite care and short-term placement

Grief is part of the bereavement process as the personality of a loved one is gradually eroded — the burden of 'ongoing bereavement'.

Social isolation occurs when demands on the carer and time constraints gradually force him/her to give up previous external activities. Attention is narrowed to the home and the patient.

Depression is not an uncommon feature in carers who, because of physical fatigue and lack of sleep caused by the patient's nocturnal activities, sink into a slough of despondency themselves.

The attending nurse should keep in mind that management of the domiciliary situation involves both the patient and the carer. The dementia management model previously outlined can be a useful means of assessing the pressures on the carer and the family, but nurses do use other approaches. Case management programmes must include assessment of the stresses and pressures on the principal carer and the need for respite care and additional assistance to reduce these. Five out of six dementia sufferers live in the community; this is a challenge for primary health care and a heavy burden on carers who are often older members of the population. Since their health may also be failing, they can be incapable of carrying this burden without major community support, which is frequently lacking.

Caring for someone with dementia stretches an individual's resources to the limit and is a far greater burden than the emotional one of caring for a physically disabled older person. This is primarily due to changes in the relationship with the dementia sufferer and behavioural changes associated with the illness. The main behavioural changes, as mentioned previously, are the result of disinhibition, deficit and maladaptation.

The loss of ability to inhibit behavioural reactions in sufferers can result in aggression, embarrassment and sexual misdemeanours. It is thought that 18 % of people with dementia are either verbally or physically aggressive, adding to the stresses experienced by the carer (Burns, 1993).

Neuropsychological deficits can create dyspraxia or lead to problems with self-care skills and a failure to carry out ordinary activities of daily living. Memory and learning problems result in disorientation, wandering and personality changes, which are particularly distressing to close relatives. All of these problems make life intolerable for the carer and when aggravated by nocturnal and daytime wandering, and incontinence, create a highly stressful situation. If they cannot be ameliorated or cured, home care will become impracticable and institutionalisation will be necessary. Efforts to delay this are usually in the best interests of the patient, but may not be so well received by an overburdened, caring relative. Their feelings, thoughts and attitudes, resilience and physical health must be considered in each step of management planning.

Five factors have been labelled as problem areas (Gilleard, 1984):

- Dependency
- Disturbance
- Disability
- Demand
- Wandering

Carers' most frequent complaint is that patients cannot be left alone, even for a short time (Askham, 1990). They wander incessantly about the house, cannot continue conversations, disrupt personal and social life, are not safe inside or outside on their own and are often incontinent.

Studies have shown that 14% of carers have significant levels of clinical depression and 33% score high in terms of psychiatric disorder on general health questionnaires. The general health of carers is poorer than that of control groups of non-caring subjects and carers are more likely to have chronic illness. Female carers experience more nervous strain than male carers, with higher levels of depression and lower morale. Male carers are more likely to be offered formal services than female carers. Daughter carers are mainly middle-aged and usually have other roles with various responsibilities for their own children. Poor previous familial relationships resulting in resentment and hostility make it unlikely that the carer will manage in the new dependent relationship. However, carers who are able to maintain positive feelings towards their dementing relatives have a lower level of perceived strain and a greater commitment to caring (Miller 1993).

Carers often feel that their role is unrecognised. Most nurses are already aware of the signs and symptoms of stress and most will employ previously learned coping strategies. The nurse's role includes care-giving for both carer and patient, and care-giving involves a comprehensive knowledge of the local and national support systems available to the carer, and referral processes that can be utilised. Issues to be addressed in a careful assessment (Martin, 1994) by the nurse include:

- The financial implications
- External factors of the spouse's own employment
- The carer's personal health and circumstances
- Other family demands
- Premorbid relationships between the carer and the dementing person
- How the carer is coping with the ongoing bereavement process
- What are the carer's coping skills?
- Is the carer claiming appropriate financial support from the state?

Stress can be reduced in carers by providing good information. The current emphasis on community care of dementing patients seems likely to continue. Its success depends very largely on the efforts of voluntary care-givers. They have a central role in supporting people with dementia. However, they may experience psychological burdens, emotional stress and ill health as a result of their involvement. The stresses and strains of caring are influenced by a number of factors, such as:

- The carer's premorbid relationship with the dementia sufferer
- The carer's interpretation of care-giving is interpreted by the carer
- The amount of informal support provided

The psychological burden of caring can be diminished by good family and friend support, and development of the carer's coping strategies and abilities. A wide range of formal support services are available to carers from social work departments and health services. These include: home helps, Meals on Wheels, laundry services, occupational therapy and the provision of respite and day care. These services enable the carer to continue functioning, as well as improving quality of life for both the carer and the dementia sufferer.

Leven (1986) found that carers reported less stress and strain when there was greater formal support even if they were not satisfied with the quantity and quality of the services provided. Gilhouly (1984) also showed that there was a positive relationship between carer morale and home help services and visits from the community nurse.

A similar pattern of benefit relates to respite care. Where respite programmes are in place, carers report improvements in their physical and mental wellbeing and an increased confidence in their ability to continue care-giving support (Burdz, 1988). District nurses working in this capacity should, however, endeavour to promote the carer's own support systems with family and friends to enhance the benefits of formal input from the State. Support agencies can also play a major part in offering respite care and support, e.g. Crossroads, and the voluntary associations (see list page 136 and Appendix).

The attending nurse must be very aware of the inner demands made on the carer. Satisfying the emotional needs of a dementia sufferer and coping with the restrictions of both providing physical care and assuming responsibility for the patient can have a profound effect on the carer's life. The first overt problem encountered is the stress generated when the problem is diagnosed. There may follow years of frustration and worsening relationships, but with the initial diagnosis there is often an unmet need for information on what the family and carer can expect in the future. To lessen the emotional impact of a diagnosis of dementia, relatives may deny the diagnosis and attribute the health disorder to a more minor condition, such as poorer sight or hearing, and may believe that the patient will be different from other sufferers and recover.

Once the disease is well established and progressive, family members often feel a sense of loss and ongoing bereavement. They feel that the person they once knew is already dead, even though still physically present. Green (1979) studied stress in carers and found that there were two classes of behaviour disturbance which were particularly difficult for carers to tolerate. One was withdrawn behaviour in the demented person, who is silent and does not interact with family members. The personal stress felt by carers arose from their feeling unable to cope, being depressed and also feeling that their own health was being undermined. The other form of behaviour disturbance which carers found difficulty in tolerating was unstable mood. If patients were moody, angry and accusing, relatives reacted negatively towards them. They felt angry, frustrated and embarrassed by the demented person. Inappropriate urinating, faecal incontinence and faecal smearing also created major problems for the carer.

Carers felt that a common factor in all their difficulties, was the demand on their time. Eighty per cent of the demented live within the community but there are hidden costs of home care which fall mainly on the carer. It has been calculated that home care, including nursing and medical and social input, always costs less than nursing home or hospital care. However, the carers pay an emotional cost and frequently suffer health problems as a result of coping with the burden.

What can be done to reduce stress in carers?

It is vital to provide adequate information. Zarit (1986) states that it is essential to give people accurate information, for this helps to alleviate the sense of crisis brought on by the family's fears concerning various aspects of the disease. Many problems that families experience with dementing patients arise from their lack of knowledge on what to do or how to respond to the changes in their relatives. Giving them adequate information puts these problems into a 'workable prospective'.

Information can be both verbal and written, but initially it is always wise to check that the carer wants more information about the disease process. Information about available services can be crucial in helping carers and reducing stress, and it is mandatory for the nurse to develop the knowledge base to meet this need. The community nurse should be aware of possible supportive contacts through the multidisciplinary team or outside agencies, with the social work management team and with voluntary support groups. Information on the Alzheimer's Association support groups, other volunteer groups, aid agencies and respite facilities should be given.

Current knowledge of the system places nurses in an ideal position to facilitate and promote support. They can also encourage medical assessment for the person with dementia and suggest a health check for the carer. It is always useful to have the carers list, in order, which problems they wish considered, and the nurse should attempt to respect their priorities. The nurse can promote the communication strategies discussed in chapter 6.

If these communication techniques are used by the family and carers, they can improve understanding between the patient and the family. Important aids to communication are simple eye language, eye contact, provision of simple tasks, time to process messages and cues and prompts where appropriate. The carer must share in the structuring of the behaviour management plan, be encouraged to provide a calm supportive atmosphere, avoid confrontation, and establish regular routines of activities of daily living for the patient.

The nurse can also encourage uptake and training programmes for carers. Many carers will refuse help but they must be encouraged to take up attendance allowances and seek additional help, and the nurse, as a key person, must keep in contact with the carer to offer continued help and guidance as the disease progresses.

Many early dementing patients live on their own and it is known that approximately 80% of elderly people using home care services are aged 75 years and over. Two-thirds are female, and

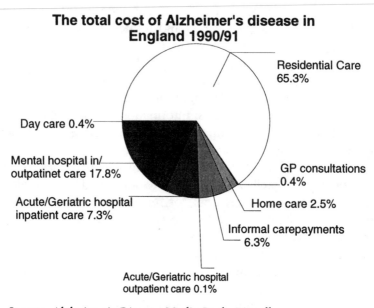

The total cost of Alzheimer's disease in England 1990/91

Residential Care 65.3%

Day care 0.4%

Mental hospital in/outpatinet care 17.8%

Acute/Geriatric hospital inpatient care 7.3%

GP consultations 0.4%

Home care 2.5%

Informal carepayments 6.3%

Acute/Geriatric hospital outpatient care 0.1%

Source: Alzheimer's Disease Media Pack, Magellan Communications (Gray and Fenn, 1993)

half of those using the services are female and aged over 75. Perhaps a quarter of this latter group will be dementing patients and it is imperative that the nurse ensures that the provision of services has been fully explored and addressed by members of the multidisciplinary team.

The former attendance allowance was replaced by the disabled living allowance (DLA) in April 1992. Again, it is important that carers take advantage of this service and apply for daytime financial support or 24-hour care. The majority of carers of dementing patients suffer from interrupted night-time sleep and are entitled to the 24-hour care allowance. These allowances are payable to anyone who requires care by another person because of mental or physical disability, and can be used to buy in additional help by day or night.

Day centre and respite care provision should be considered in the early stages, if only to ensure that the patient is on the waiting list. It is vital for these facilities to be set up early, if the carer's involvement is to be long term. Day centres are run by social services and voluntary organisations, and the day hospitals by local health authorities. Day care, when offered early to a patient, allows him/her to adapt better and to benefit more from the experience. It offers a change of scene and a new focus of interest as well as a range of stimulating activities. It ensures that carers have time completely free from any obligation to the patient, and allows them to shop, socialise and maintain some conventional routines for themselves.

10
Patient safety in the community

Potential hazards

A constant source of concern for carers is the risk of hazard and **accidents** to the dementing relative, occurring in the home or in the neighbourhood of the home. Many patients with dementia are elderly and already at added risk. A balance and compromise has to be organised whereby the patient's freedom is not overly curtailed. The risk of minor mishaps, accidents and falls has to be accepted. This is the price to be paid for functional orientated nursing care.

Particular aids to be considered are handrails, bath aids and toilet aids. The occupational therapist can advise on mechanical aids and ways of making the home safer. Poor lighting is a source of confusion and accidents which should be addressed. Obviously, there has to be close supervision of medications; these may have to be physically provided by a nurse, relative or neighbour rather than using conventional container medication on the assumption that the patient will take medication on written instructions.

Smoking creates an additional risk of fire hazard and is a difficult problem to resolve. Some method of supervision is advisable. Smoke detectors must be installed, but some risk remains if smokers insist on smoking in bed at night.

Alcohol can also create problems for dementing patients. It can cause further confusion and, if taken with medication, is likely to cause interactions, such as over-sedation or over-agitation.

Driving is a major concern in the early dement and the nurse must ensure that the patient abstains from driving. Several studies have shown conclusively that, even in early dementia, there is impaired judgment and orientation in drivers, who are more likely to have an accident than elders in their peer group who are free from dementia. There is a statutory obligation for this class of driver to be reported to the Vehicle Licensing Authority if they do not abstain from driving.

Cooking and open fires remain hazards. The risk from open fires can be contained to some extent by the use of fixed guards, but cooking should be undertaken by the attending relative.

Hypothermia is always a risk for elderly patients, especially in the winter months, but is a particular risk for dementing patients who are unaware of the need for extra heating.

Carers may need advice on **maintaining patient hygiene** in terms of bathing and continence aids and the occupational therapist should be approached for early advice in assessing these needs.

Nursing stresses

Caring for the carer and the patient can be a stressful experience for the attending nurse. This has to be recognised and problems should be shared with the nurse manager, GP or other team members. The load should not be carried alone. There are many responsibilities, and a broad awareness of the organisations and facilities which can support all those involved is needed. The nurse should keep in mind that he/she is part of the primary care team and an extended multidisciplinary team, all of whom are involved in the management of these patients. There must be a willingness to recognise the point at which others should be involved and the GP, in particular, should be advised of a change in patient status. Referral to specialists for medical, psychiatric and other services is an important decision-making consideration. Timing is often crucial and is ideally best determined in conference with other members of the team.

The primary care team

The primary care team may include occupational therapist, clinical psychologist, community psychiatric worker, health visitor, social worker and the patient's own doctor. Several voluntary agencies may be involved. Overall, clinical responsibility remains with the GP as long as the patient lives at home. Geriatricians and other clinicians may become responsible for managing the physical decline, whereas psychiatrists and psychogeriatricians will be primarily involved with the psychological decline, especially when psychiatric disease dominates in the final stages of AD. With a large number of health professionals possibly involved, there is a real risk that the patient will fall between stools and not receive the optimal attention he/she deserves. This is an important consideration for the attending nurse to keep in mind.

Carer abuse of the dementing patient

Abuse control

The majority of dementia sufferers are cared for by the family members, such as elderly spouses, daughters and daughters-in-law. Exhaustion, exasperation, anger, isolation, and variable availability and quality of service input can take carers to the brink of their own psychological capacity. As much as 50% of all carers risk psychiatric illness (Office of Population Censuses and Surveys, 1988) and many become overdependent on alcohol and drugs. It is, therefore, not surprising that many carers begin to abuse their charges.

Studies in the USA suggest that between 2 and 10% of the elderly are at risk of abuse and a considerable number of these will be dementing patients. Elderly abuse appears to occur regardless of social class or ethnic background. The majority of victims are female and the gender of the abuser is related to the type of abuse. A high proportion of spouse abuse involves women abusing husbands. Males appear to be more likely to cause physical abuse to the dementing patient, whereas females are more likely to neglect their care duties.

Nurses should be awake to the possibilities of abuse of dementing patients. Abuse has been defined as follows:

1   Neglect — the deprivation of ordinary everyday requirements, such as food and warmth

2   Psychological — intimidation, humiliation, embarrassment and dehumanisation

3   Financial — carer or neighbour persuades the person with dementia to sign over pension, etc

4   Isolation — either restraint or confinement away from normal social interactions

5   Physical assault — hitting and beating

6   Over-sedation with drugs or deprivation of prescribed drugs

Positive signs of patient wellbeing

It is not always easy to determine whether a mentally ill patient with communication difficulties is enoying any quality of life. Many of the normal pointers to wellbeing will be absent in behaviour or distorted so that they may be hard to interpret. Some features shown by aphasic and mute patients can point towards relative contentment:

Relaxation — requests are met congenially and willingly

Sensitivity to the needs of others — the patient is not stubborn and self-centred

Humour — expression and conduct indicate a sense of fun

Helpfulness — asked for and unrequested aid proferred

Pleasure — countenance and actions infer enjoyment

Affection — demonstrated by gesture, facial expression and non-verbal behaviour

Emotional expression — varying responses in appropriate ways

Acceptance of others and willingness to participate in social interaction

Creativity — innovative behaviour; artistic expression

Assertiveness without being self-centred or attention-seeking

Initiation of social contact

Features which diminish the self-worth of the demented patient

Some carers either deliberately or accidently diminish the psychological status of their charges by:

Disempowerment —the patients is refused the option of decision-taking

Infantalisation — the patient is treated like a baby

Stigmatisation — the patient is overtly labelled as being mad, etc

Banishment — the patient is excluded from family living situations or kept away from people in a room

Intimidation — the patient is threatened verbally or physically or abused

Invalidation — social interactions and observations are negated by the carer

Objectification — the patient is treated as an object, kept clean and safe but given no respect as a human being

Treachery — misuse of the patient's funds, property or body

Nurses should be aware of the possibilities of such conduct in carers and keep in mind that some of these features can easily be adopted in continuing nursing care, when time is at a premium, behaviour is troublesome and beneficial therapeutic endeavour is limited (Archibald, 1995).

Factors which suggest that abuse may be likely, imminent or existing

- Marked behaviour disorder, disinhibition or aggression in a patient
- Reports of falls, minor injuries, burns, bite marks, evidence of neglect and malnutrition in the patient
- Expressive and receptive dysphasia in a patient

If the elderly carer was abused as a child, there is strong research evidence that he/she will react abusively in adulthood. Sometimes the carer is making overfrequent visits to the GP, which may be a *cri de coeur*. The attending nurse must keep the possibility in mind, but the risk must also be kept in proportion. The majority of carers are highly committed to their responsibilities and perform a very good job of caring for the demented. Some abuse results from the inadequacy of state support systems in meeting needs.

The nurse may find difficulties in identifying abuse because:

- The abuser may restrict access
- The abuser may insist on being present during conversation with the patient
- The abused person may be dependent on the carer and will therefore be reluctant to report abuse
- The patient may feel guilty about sexual abuse

The nurse has a crucial role to play in the prevention of abuse by being aware of the risk factors, regularly assessing the dementing patient and offering early intervention to reduce stress in the carer. Early input of social and health services may reduce the pressure on the carer. Referral to appropriate services may also counterbalance the risk of financial abuse, which is the most common form of abuse by carers and other interested parties.

The nurse should be prepared to listen to what the person with dementia has to say on the subject. Although they may not be able to express themselves clearly and inform the nurse that they are being abused, they may give clues such as 'he keeps touching me' or 'he comes to me at night'. By keeping a close eye on medication compliance and supplies, the nurse can also control any drug mismanagement. Anticipatory management early in the disease process may prepare and guide carers as the patient deteriorates, helping them to maintain coping abilities in a continuing stressful situation.

Refusal of service

The nurse may become involved when the carer refuses to accept services and, equally, may find it necessary to help change the patient's attitude when he/she is rigorously refusing to accept caring input. Risks, choices and options must be fully explored and balanced. In such instances, out-of-hours crisis intervention will be needed at a time when there will be limited social service input. This cannot be avoided when there is a failure to realistically accept offered services, and the nurse may be forced to accept frustration when having to cope with a potentially avoidable situation. In some cases, the only acceptable solution is for the nurse to continue to review the situation and try to change entrenched attitudes.

Refusal to allow patients to enter residential care should prompt the nurse to consider the possibility that some form of abuse is being perpetrated or that there is some financial advantage to the carer if the patient remains in the home. Equally, carers often become overcommitted to their charges and may need to be counselled and encouraged to accept the offered care. Compulsory procedures are possible in cases of demented patients living on their own, but these should be avoided until every other option has been explored.

Support organisations

There are many voluntary associations involved in the support of demented patients and their carers. Information is available from:

- The Carer's National Association
- Alzheimer's Disease Society
- Age Concern
- British Association for Services to the Elderly
- Alzheimer's Scotland (Action on Dementia (ASAD))

Day hospital support for carers and patients

Limited periods of a day or short-term breaks can be organised to ease the strain on carers and optimise care for the patient.

The aims of the hospital nurse caring for patients in the short term are to:

1   Maintain or increase patients' independence

2   Ensure patient comfort and support carers

3   Facilitate the patients' return home by trying to alter patient behaviours which carers have found stressful

Leven (1983) reported that carers experienced a reduction in anxiety and an increase in their ability to cope with a sick family member as a result of:

1   Nurses listening to carers with unconditional acceptance of their feelings

2   Short breaks from the sick family member provided by sitter service, day hospital or respite care

Appendix

Societies and associations

Age Concern England, Astral House, 1268 London Road, London, SW16 4ER, Tel: 01 81 679 8000
>   **Aims**: A centre of policy, research, information and social advocacy on all subjects regarding the welfare of elderly people. Local Age Concern groups throughout the UK help with provision of day centres, Meals-on-Wheels, etc.

Age Concern Scotland, 54A Fountainbridge, Edinburgh, EH3 9PT

Alzheimer's Disease Society, Gordon House, 10 Greencoat Place, London, SW1P 1PH, Tel: 01 71 306 0606
>   **Aims**: To support families and professionals carinf someone with Alzheimer's disease or other forms of dementia. Booklist and information leaflets on the disease, its diagnosis and management are available.

Alzheimer's Scotland — Action on Dementia, 8 Hill Street, Edinburgh, Scotland, EH2 3JZ, Tel: 01 31 225 1453
>   **Aims**: To support Scottish families and professionals caring for someone with Alzheimer's disease or other forms of dementia. Information leaflets on many aspects of dementia and home care are available.

British Association for Services to the Elderly (BASE), 119 Hassell Street, Newcastle-under-Lyme, Staffordshire, ST5 1AX, Tel: 01 782 661033

> **Aims**: Organises study days and training courses for those running services to the elderly.

Carers National Association, 29 Chilworth Mews, London, W2 3RG, Tel: 01 71 724 7776

> **Aims**: Advice and information to people looking after ill, disabled or elderly frail relatives or friends at home. Branches and self help groups.

Continuing Care at Home Association (CONCAH), 54 Glasshouse Lane, Countess Wear, Exeter, EX2 7BU

> **Aims**: To improve the relief of disabled or sick people confined to their homes, and to improve the knowledge and understanding of their carers.

Dementia Services Development Centre, University of Stirling, Stirling, Scotland, FK9 4CA, Tel: 01 786 467744

> **Aims**: Maintain a library of 3,500 books which is avialable to statutory charities. Will supply information and advice to health board staff. Economically priced books on practical aspects of dementia management.

Health Matters, 47A Fleet Street, Swindon, SN1 1RE, Tel: 01 793 618 558

> **Aims**: Works with self-help groups, carers and health service professionals, provides information on local sources of help, runs training courses, undertakes research, promotes a consumer voice in the planning of health services.

Help the Aged, 16-18 St James Walk, London, EC1R 0BE, Tel: 01 71 253 0253

    Aims: To improve the quality of life of elderly people, particularly those who are frail, isolated or poor. To identify needs by raising public awareness and promote and develop aid programmes.

Invalid Care Allowance Unit, Pallatine House, Lancaster Road, Preston, PR1 1NS, Tel: 01 253 856 123

    Aims: Information on invalid care allowance only.

Medic Alert Foundation, 12 Bridge Wharf, 156 Caledonian Road, London, N1 8BR.

MINI-MENTAL STATE EXAMINATION (MMSE)

Record response to each question

ORIENTATION

1. Year, Month, Day, Date, Season   /5

2. Country, County (District), Town,   /5
    Hospital, Ward (Room)
    REGISTRATION

3. Examiner names three objects   /3
    (e.g. Orange, Ball, Key).
    Patient asked to repeat the three
    names.
    Score one for each correct answer
    Then ask patient to repeat the names three times.

ATTENTION

4. Subtract 7 from 100, and 7 from the result etc.
    Stop after 5 (100, 93, 86, 79, 72, 65)
    (Do not correct if errors made)

    (Alternatively spell WORLD backwards: DLROW)

    Score the best performance on either task   /5
    RECALL

5. Ask for the names of the three objects   /3
    learned earlier
    LANGUAGE

6. Name a pencil and a watch   /2

7. Repeat "No ifs, ands or buts"   /1

8. Give a three stage command.Score one
    for each stage,
    (e.g. "Take this piece of paper in your
    left hand,

fold it in half, and place it on the ground") /3

9. Ask patient to read and obey a written command on a piece of paper
    "CLOSE YOUR EYES"   /1

10.

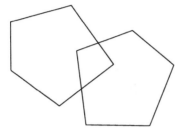

Ask patient to write a sentence. Score if sensible, has a subject and a verb

COPYING

11. Ask patient to copy intersecting pentagons   /1

   TOTAL SCORE   /30

This test is said to be subject to variation based on cultural, educational and socioeconomic status>

Standard Cut Off: 24 or more = Normal; 23 or less = Impaired

Age related Cut Off: 40s   N = 29 or more
                         50s   N = 28 or more
                         60s   N = 28 or more
                         70s   N = 28 or more
                         80s   N = 26 or more

Less than 10 years of full time education: three extra errors allowed

HACHINSKI ISCHAEMIC SCORE

A score of 4 or less is taken to be suggestive of AD

A score of 7 or more suggests VAD

Clinical date (History or Clinical sign)	Ischaemia score
Abrupt onset	2
Fluctuating course	1
Nocturnal confusion	1
Relative preservation of personality	1
Depression	1
Somatic complaints	1
Emotional incontinence	1
History of hypertension	1
History of strokes	2
Evidence of atherosclerosis	1
Focal neurological symptoms	2
Focal neurological signs	2
Stepwise deterioration	1

Patient Name/Identification _____

HAMILTON PSYCHIATRIC RATING SCALE FOR DEPRESSION (HAM–D)

INVESTIGATOR _____ Date of Visit _____

Details of how to score each item are explained in the guidelines which can be found on the card in the inside pocket at the front of this record book

1.	DEPRESSED MOOD	0-4		12.	SOMATIC SYMPTOMS GASTROINTESTINAL	0-2
2.	FEELINGS OF GUILT	0-4		13.	SOMATIC SYMPTOMS GENERAL	0-2
3.	SUICIDE	0-4		14.	GENITAL SYMPTOMS	0-4
4.	INSOMNIA: EARLY	0-2		15.	HYPOCHONDRIASIS	0-2
5.	INSOMNIA: MIDDLE	0-2		16.	LOSS OF WEIGHT	0-2
6.	INSOMNIA: LATE	0-2		17.	INSIGHT (when in fact ill)	
7.	WORK AND ACTIVITIES	0-4			Total Score of first 17 items	_____
8.	RETARDATION	0-4		18.	DIURNAL VARIATION	0-2
9.	AGITATION	0-4			If present, please indicate whether symptoms are worse in the morning or evening Worse in morning Worse in evening	
10.	ANXIETY: PSYCHIC	0-4		19.	DEREAISATION & DEPERSONALISATION	0-4
11.	ANXIETY: SOMATIC	0-4		20.	PARANOID SYMPTOMS	0-4
				21.	OBSESSIONAL SYMPTOMS	0-2

Score of 17 or more - Depression likely

Activities of Daily Living Scale

		before illness					
BARTHEL INDEX	Surname . . . . Forename(s) . . . . Sex . . . . Date of Birth Address						
Date of Examination		before illness					
BOWELS[1]	0 Incontinent 1 Occasional accident (once a week) 2 Continent						
BLADDER[2]	0 Incontinent 1 Occasional accident (once per 24hrs) 2 Continent (for more than 7 days)						
GROOMING[3]	0 Needs help with personal care 1 Independent (implements provided)						
TOILETUSE[4]	0 Dependent 1 Needs some help 2 Independent						
FEEDING[5]	0 Unable 1 Needs help (cutting spreading etc) 2 Independent (food within reach)						
TRANSFER[6]	0 Unable – no sitting balance 1 Major help (physical, 1 or 2 people) 2 Minor help (verbal or physical) 3 Independent						
MOBILITY[7]	0 Immobile 1 Wheelchair independent 2 Walks with help of one person 3 Independent						
DRESSING[8]	0 Dpendent 1 Needs help but can do half unaided 2 Independent (incl buttons, zips, laces)						
STAIRS[9]	0 Unable 1 Needs help (verbal or physical) 2 Independent up and down						
BATHING[10]	0 Dependent 1 Independent						
TOTAL SCORE (best = 20, worst = 0)							

OVER – 75s ASSESSMENT PROFILE

NAME	NAME AND RELATIONSHIP OF CARING RELATIVE OR NEXT OF KIN:
CIVIL STATUS M/S/W/D	NAME ....
DATE OF BIRTH	ADDRESS.................................
ADDRESS...............................	....
....	....
TELEPHONE	....
TYPE OF HOUSING	TELEPHONE ....

SERVICES NEEDED: R = Required, P = Provided, D = Discontinued, Ref = Refused

DATE OF REVIEW										
CHIROPODY										
DAY HOSPITAL										
DENTAL CARE										
OPTICIAN										
AUDIOMETRY										
DISTRICT NURSE										
HEALTH VISITOR										
SOCIAL WORKER										
HOME HELP										
HOSPITAL										
HOUSING										
MEDICAL EMERGENCY CARE SERVICE										
MEALS ON WHEELS										
OT										
OTHERS ( )										

ACTIVIES OF DAILY LIVING:

DATE											
SCORE	HOUSEHOLD										
0.	Fully Independent										
1.	Friend or relative lives with them										
2.	Friend or relative visits regularly										
3.	Dependent on social services										
4.	Dependent on community nurses etc										

5.	Combination										
	Sub-totals										
BEREAVEMENT OF SPOUSE OR SIBLING											
0.	None										
1.	Less than 2 years										
2.	Less than 6 months										
	Sub-totals										
SCORE	**HOUSING**										
0.	No problems										
1.	Too big										
2.	Too many stairs or similar										
4.	Damp or poor condition of housing										
5.	Multiple housing problems										
	Sub-totals										
WARMTH											
0.	Adequate										
3.	Barely adequate										
5.	Inadequate										
	Sub-totals										
MOBILITY											
0.	Full mobility										
2.	Mobile with aids										
4.	Housebound										
5.	Bed or chairbound										
	Sub-totals										
CONTINENCE											
0.	Fully continent										
2.	Stress incontinence or urgency										
4.	Day/night incontinence										
5.	Incontinent of urine and faeces										
	Sub-totals										

VISION											
0.	Satisfactory										
1.	Uses vision aid										
3.	Partially sighted										
5.	Blind										
	Sub-totals										
HEARING											
0.	No noticeable loss										
1.	Satisfactory with hearing aid										
3.	Unsatisfactory with/without aid										
5.	Total deafness										
	Sub-totals										
HYGIENE											
0.	Satisfactory										
1.	Satisfactory with aids										
3.	Bath or shower with assistance										
4.	Dirty or unkempt										
	Sub-totals										
DIET											
0.	Satisfactory										
1.	Satisfactory with supplied meals										
3.	Deficient										
	Sub-totals										

DATE											
SCORE	WEIGHT										
0.	Normal										
2.	Moderately obese										
4.	Underweight/obese										
5.	Very underweight/very obese										
	Sub-totals										

SLEEP											
0.	Sleeps well without sedation										
2.	Disturbed sleep										
3.	Sleeps well with sedation										
	Sub-totals										
EMOTIONAL ASSESSMENT											
0.	No problems										
2.	Discontented										
4.	Very unhappy										
	Sub-totals										

The Carer	Comments:
Gender	
Health Status	
Psychological Status	
Coping Status	
Family Support	
Network Support	
Special Needs	
Evidence of Abuse	

MEDICAL ASSESSMENT: (At each assesment score:
0 = no symptoms to 5 = severe symptoms) (Scored by GP)

DATE											
1.	CARDIOVASCULAR										
2.	ENDOCRINE										
3.	GASTROINTESTINAL										
4.	GENITOURINARY										
5.	LOCOMOTOR										
6.	MEMORY LOSS										
7.	NERVOUS SYSTEM										

8.	PSYCHIATRIC										
9.	RESPIRATORY										
10.	SKIN										
	SCORE TOTALS										
	MEDICAL										
	DAILY LIVING										
	CUMULATIVE SCORE										
	PATIENT'S INITIALS (if required)										

MENTAL STATUS:

INSTRUCTIONS:

Ask questions 1-9 in this list and record all errors

Ask question 4A only if patient does not have a telephone

Record the total number of errors based on 9 questions.

RESULTS:

0-2 errors, intact intellectual function

3-4 errors, mild intellectual impairment

5-7 errors, moderate intellectual impairment

8-9 errors, severe intellectual impairment

DATE											
1.	What is the date today? (d-m-y)										
2.	What day of the week is it?										
3.	What is the name of this place?										
4.	What is your telephone number?										
4A.	What is your street address? (ask only if no telephone)										
5.	How old are you?										
6.	When were you born? (d-m-y)										
7.	Who is the Prime Minister now?										
8.	What was your mother's maiden name										
9.	Take 3 away from 20 and keep taking 3 from each new number you get, all the way down										
	TOTAL ERRORS										

MEDICATION/MEDICAL NEEDS:

	DATE	PRODUCT	DOSE	NOTES
1.				
2.				
3.				
4.				
5.				
6.				
7.				

ABBREVIATED MENTAL TEST SCORE

- Age
- Time (to nearest hour)
- Address for recall at the end of the test, e.g. 42 West Street. This should be repeated by the patient to ensure that it has been heard correctly
- Year
- Name of hospital
- Recognition of two persons, e.g. doctor, nurse
- Date of birth
- Year of First World War
- Name of present monarch
- Count backwards from 20

Each question scores one mark. Scores below 7 indicate the possibility of cognitive impairment.

References

Alzheimer A (1909). A Peculiar Disease of the Cerebral Cortex, *Allg Z Psychiatry*, **64**, 146

Allan K (1994). *Wandering*, Dementia Services Development Centre, University of Stirling

Annon J (1976). The PLISST Model, *J Sex Educ Ther*, **2**, 1–15

Archibald C (1994). *Sexuality and Dementia*, Dementia Services Development Centre, University of Stirling.

Archibald C, Chapman A and Weaks D (1995). *A practice guide for community nurses*, Dementia Services Development Centre, University of Stirling

Armstrong-Esther C and Browne K (1986). *J Adv Nurs Care*, **11**, 379–87

Askham J and Thompson C (1990). *Dementia and Home Care*, Age Concern Institute of Gerontology, Research Paper 104

Blessed G, Tomlinson B and Roth M (1968). Associations between Quantitative Measures of Dementia and Senile Change in the Cerebral Grey Matter of Elderly Subjects, *B J Psych*, **114**, 797–811.

Brooking J (1986). Dementia and Confusion in the Elderly, in Reagen S (ed), *Nursing Elderly People*, Churchill Livingstone, Edinburgh.

Brook P, Degun G and Mather M (1975). Reality Orientation — A Controlled Study, *B J Psych*, **127**, 42–45.

Butler R (1963). The Life Review — Interpretation of Reminiscence in the Aged, *Psych*, **26**, 65–76.

Burnside I (ed) (1981). *Nursing and the Aged, 2nd edn*, McGraw Hill, New York.

Bliwise D (1994). What is Sundowning, *J A G S*, **42**, 1001–11.

Burns A and Levy R (1993). *Dementia*, Chapman, London.

Burdz M and Eaton W (1988). Effect of Respite Care on Dementia and Non-Dementia Patients and Caregivers, *Psych & Ageing*, **3**, 38–42.

Carr J and Marshall M (1993). Innovations in Longstay Care in People with Dementia, review in *Clin Geront*, **3**, 157–167.

Chapman A and Marshall M (eds) (1993). *Dementia: new skills for social workers*, Kingsley, London

Evers H (1982). Professional Practice in Patient Care, *Ageing in Soc*, **2**, 57–75.

Editorial (1994). Wondering about the Wanders, *Lancet*, 1237–8.

Folstein M, Folstein S and McHugh P (1975). Mini-Mental State, *J Psych Res*, **12**, 189–98.

Feil N (1982). *Validation; The Feil Method*, Feil Productions, Cleveland, Ohio.

FVHB (1992). *Estimates of Dementia*, Public Health Medicine Health Information Note 8

Gibson F (1994). Reading around reminiscence, *J Dem Care*, **2**, 3, 24–5.

Gibson F (1994). *Reminiscence and Recall Guide to Good Practice*, Age Concern, London.

Gilleard C (1984). *Living with dementia*, Croom Helm, London.

Gilhooly M (1984). The impact of care-giving on carers, *Br J Med Psychol*, **54**, 35–44.

Green J and Timbury G A (1979). A geriatric psychiatric day hospital service, *Age & Ageing*, **8**, 49–53.

Gray A (1993). Alzheimer's Disease: The burden of the illness in England, *Health Trends*, **25**, 1, 31–37.

Hamilton M (1960). A Rating Scare for Depression, *J Neurol Neurosurg & Psych*, **22**, 56–62.

Hachinsky V, Lassen N and Marshall J (1994). Multi-infarct Dementia; a cause of mental deterioration in the Elderly, *Lancet*, **2**, 207–9.

Henderson A (1988). Risk Factors for Alzheimer's Disease — A Review, *Acta Psychiat Scand*, **78**, 257–75.

Holden N (1990). *Reality Orientation, Working with Dementia*, Wilmslow Press, Bicester.

Henderson V, Mack W and Williams B (1989). Spatial disorientation in Alzheimer's Disease 1981, *Arch Neurol*, **46**, 391–4.

Illiffe S, Mitchley S *et al* (1994). Evaluation of Brief Screening Instruments for Dementia, Depression in General Practice, *Br J G P*, 503–7.

Janssen J and Gibberson D (1988). Remotivation Therapy, *J Gerontol Nurs*, **14** (6), 31–34.

Jorm A and Korten A (1988). A Method of Calculating Prognostic Increase in Number of Dementia Sufferers, *Aust & NZ J Psych*, **22**, 183–9.

Jorm A, Korten A and Henderson A (1987). Prevalence of Dementia, *Acta Psychiat Scand*, **766**, 466–479.

Keady J (1994). Younger Onset Dementia, *J Adv Nurs*, **19**, 659–669.

Kellet J (1989). Dementia and the Elderly, *Br Med J*, 934.

Kitwood T (1989). Discover the person not the disease, *J Dement Care*, **1**, Nov, 16–17

Kitwood T and Bredin K (1992). A New Approach to Evaluation of Dementia Care, *J Adv Health & Nurs Care*, **1**, 5, 41–60.

Kitwood T (1993). Towards a theory of dementia care: The interpersonal process, *Age Soc*, **13**, 51–67

Klerk Rubin V (1994). How Validation is Misunderstood, *J Dem Care*, **2**, 2, 14–16.

Lawton M and Brody E (1969). Assessment of Older People, *Gerontol*, **9**, 9, 179–86.

Levin E, Sinclair I and Gorback P (1983). *The Supporters of Confused Elderly Persons at Home*, Nat Institute Society Work, London.

McIntosh I (1988). Geriatric Surveillance & Management: Using a Two-Year Trained Nurse, *Scot Med*, **5**, 332–3.

McIntosh I (1990). Screening the over 75s, *Geriatrix J A R D*, **3.4,** 6–7

McIntosh I and Young M (1990). An over 75s assessment checklist, *Ger Med*, **Mar, Suppl1**.

McIntosh I (1993). Should we screen the elderly, *Med Monit*, **7 June**, 32.

McIntosh I and Power K (1993). Elderly peoples' views of annual screening assessment, *J R C G P*, **43**, 370, 189–193.

McLennan J, Murdoch P and McIntosh I (1993). *Dementia Touches Everyone — a GP guide*, Dementia Services Development Centre, University of Stirling, Stirling

McShane R (1994). Wellbeing and Wandering, *J Dem Care*, **2**, 5, 24–5.

McShane R, Hope T and Wilkinson J (1994). Tracking Patients who Wander, *Lancet*, **343**, 1274.

Marshall M (1993). Wandering is a Myth, *J Dem Care*, **1**, 6, 11.

Martin C, Pickles A and Wattis J (1994). Helping Carers Cope with Withdrawn Behaviour, *Ger Med*, **April**, 23.

Masterson A (1993). Special Skills for Future Needs, *J Dem Care*, **1**, 6, 14.

Miller E and Morris K (1993). *The Psychology of Dementia*, Wiley Press, Chichester.

Morris R and Baddeby A (1988). Primary and Working Memory in Alzheimer's Type Dementia, *J Clin Exp Neuropsych*, **10**, 279–296.

Neri L and Hewitt D (1991). Aluminium Alzheimer's Disease and Drinking Water, *Lancet*, 38–90.

Orrell M, Howard R, Payne A *et al* (1992). Differentiation between Organic and Functional Psychiatric Illness in the Elderly, *Intl J Ger Psych*, **7**, 263–75.

Pattie A and Gillard C (1981). *Manual of Clifton Assessment Procedures (CAPE)*, Hodder Stoughton, Kent.

Rapp M, Flint A *et al* (1992). Behaviour Disturbance in Demented Elderly, *Can J Psych*, **37**, 251–57.

Rawlinson A and Brown A (1993). The Community Psychiatric Nurse, *Scott Med*, **11**, 6, 8–9.

Roger N and Logan W *et al* (1980). *The Elements of Nursing*, Churchill Livingstone, Edinburgh.

Rosen G, Terry R, Fuld D *et al* (1980). Pathological Verification of Ischaemic Score in Differentiation of Dementia, *Ann Neurol*, **7**, 486–8.

Rosen G, Mohns R and Davis K (1984). A New Rating Scale for Alzheimer's Disease, *Am J Psych*, **141** (11), 1356–64.

Roth M, Thym E *et al* (1986). Camdex — A Standardised Instrument for Diagnosing Mental Disorder in the Elderly, *Br J Psych*, **149**, 698–709.

Seaman A (1982). Effective Nursing Touch, *Ger Nurs*, **June**, 162–4.

Tobiansky R (??date??). Understanding Dementia, *J Dem Care*, **1**, 6, 26–28.

Tombaugh T and McIntyre N (1992). MMSE: A Comprehensive Review, *J A G S*, **40**, 922–35.

Watkins M (1988). Lifting the Burden, *Ger Nurs & Home Care*, **Oct**, 17–19.

Wilkieson C, McWhirter M and McIntosh I *et al* (1995). Health assessments 3 years on — Are they still of benefit, *Age & Ageing*, **24, Supp 1**.40, 16.

Wilson B (1987). *Rehabilitation of Memory*, Guildford Press, New York.

Wilson R, Bacon, Fox J *et al* (1983). Primary Memory and Secondary Memory in Dementia of Alzheimer's Type, *J Clin Neuropsych*, **5**, 337–44.

Woods R (1994). Reading around Reality Orientation, *J Dem Care*, **1**, 2, 24–25.

Zarit S, Todd P and Zarit J (1986). Subjective Burden of Husbands and Wives as Caregivers, *Gerontol*, **20**, 260–266.

Index

A

Abbreviated Mental Test
Scale 28, 36
abuse 138, 139
  financial 136
  isolation 136
  neglect 136
  over-sedation 136
  physical assault 136
  prevention 139
  psychological 136
  sexual 139
abuse control 135
accidents 133
accusation 102
action plan 68
activities of daily living 33
AD 3, 5, 6, 7, 10, 11, 13, 14, 15, 16,
  17, 28, 36, 38, 71, 72, 73, 74, 83,
  85, 121, 122
  See Also Alzheimer's disease
  clinical features 19
  See Also course of the disease
  criteria for the diagnosis 27
  early stage 17
  emotional change features 19
  insidious onset 27
  late stage 18
  middle stage 17
ADAS 36
  See Also Alzheimer's Disease
Assessment
ADL 33, 55
  See Also activities of daily living
aggression 86, 93, 102
agitation and restlessness 97
agnosia 85
AIDS 13

See Also Auto Immune Deficiency
Syndrome
alcohol 13, 133
altered sleep patterns 110
aluminium 15
Alzheimer's 1, 3, 10, 11, 24, 31, 49,
  84, 121
  memory defects 72
  onset 11
Alzheimer's Association support 129
Alzheimer's Disease Assessmen 28
Alzheimer's Disease Society 121
AMTS 28, 36
  See Also Abbreviated Mental Test
Scale
anger 99, 102
annual geriatric surveillance 16, 40,
  47
anoxia 13
anxiety 19
apathy 86, 109
aphasia 85
assertiveness 67
assessment 32, 43
  goals 43
  protocols 41
attendance allowance 130
attention-seeking 105
Auto Immune Deficiency Syndro 13
autopsy 61

B

babying 100
banishment 64, 138
BARTHEL Index 28, 37
BASDEC 37
  See Also Brief Assessment
  Schedule Dep
behavioural changes 20, 23
benign senile forgetfulness 73

bereavement process 126, 128
beta blockers 116
Binswangers Disease 13
biography 50
a biomedical model 45
Blessed Dementia Scale 36
blood count 32
blood glucose 32
boredom 104
Bradykinesia 23
brain cortex 71
Brief Assessment Schedule Dep 37

C
calcium levels 32
CAMDEX 36
CAPE
See Also Clifton Assessment
Procedure
Care
associations 35
planning 55
team 42
value 67, 68
care managers
social work 41
the carer 43, 71, 84, 89
caring for 121
carers 3, 61, 65, 66, 68, 69, 76, 82,
83, 102, 122, 124
abuse 135
community 16
daughter 125
familial 93
family 16, 91
female 125
formal 60
health 125
informal 60
male 125
needs 33
professional 93
voluntary 3
catastrophic reactions 25, 93, 98, 99
cerebral
atrophy 2
biopsy 16
infections 13
cerebrovascular disease 13

Challenging the assumptions 61
chlorpromazine 102
chromosome 12 15
chromosome 14 15
chromosome 19 15
chromosome 21 14
classical conditioning 53
Clifton Assessment Procedure 37
clinical nurse specialist 41, 47
clinical psychologist
psychiatric worker 135
cognition 11, 71
cognitive
changes 20, 22
deficiencies 71
impairment 16
losses 71
management 71
skills 71
communication 55, 85
barriers 87
guidelines 86
impasse 87
management 88
non-verbal 53, 84, 91
problems 89
skills 109
verbal 53, 84
community
liaison nurse 39
nurse 3, 41, 76, 127, 129
nurse support 4
patient safety 133
psychiatric nurse 3, 39, 76, 102
psychiatric worker 135
support 124
confabulation 74
provoked 75
spontaneous 75
confounding differential
diagnosis 16
confusion 24, 56
acute 29
continence 33
aids 119
cooking 134
coping strategies 77, 78, 125
Cortical Lewy body type 6, 9

counselling
  sexual 115
CPN
  psychiatric nurse 102
  see also: 102
  See also: community psychiatric
  nurse 102
Crossroads, 127
cues
  auditory 77
  verbal 77
cytoplasm 10

D
  DAT 9
  See Also Dementia of Alzheimer's
  type
day
  care 131
  centre 130
  hospital 82
  hospital support 140
delirium 12, 28, 29, 111
  acute 28
delusions 18, 75, 76
dementia 1-10, 13, 16, 18, 24, 26,
29-32, 34, 39-41, 43, 45-50, 52-55,
61, 62, 65-67, 69, 71, 73, 76, 81,
83, 96, 101-103, 109, 114, 116
  arteriosclerotic 6
  assessment plan 54
  care mapping 67
  carer 121
  cerebrovascular 9
  chronic 7
  confounding causes 28
  cortical vascular 13
  differential diagnosis 12
  Lewy body-type 31
  management model 124
  management of 51
  management plan 54
  mild 27, 60
  moderate 27, 60
  multi-infarct 6, 9-10, 13, 24, 31, 81
  pre-senile 7
  senile 1, 7, 62
  severe 27, 60, 75
  spouse 115

  stress management 53
  subcortical vascular 13
  vascular 9, 36
dementia
Dementia of Alzheimer's type 9
Dementia Services
demographic trends 5
depression 19, 24, 28, 29, 30, 31,
  41, 109, 111, 125
diagnosis chart 25
Diagnostic and Statistical Manual
  of Mental Disorders 27
diagnostic criteria 11
diary use 77
diazepam 102, 107
differential diagnosis 27
difficulties
  motor 53
  perceptional 53
Diffuse Lewy body disease 10
directive intervention 106
disability 125
disabled living allowance 130
disempowerment 63, 137
disinhibition 114
  frontal lobes 114
disorientation 86, 105, 124
disruptive behaviour 97
  management 93
  Sexual 93
disruptive vocal behaviour 98
district nurses 16, 40, 41
DLA
  See also: disabled living
  allowance 130
Down's syndrome 14
driving 134
drowsiness 16, 107
drug mismanagement 139
drugs 13
  major tranquillisers 102
  minor tranquillisers 102
DSM 27
  See Also Diagnostic and Statistical
  Manual of Mental Disorders
dyspraxia 124

E

EEG 38

See Also Electroencephalography

Electroencephalography 38

electrolytes 32

electronic aids 106

emotional changes 22

emotional problem

  aggression 123

  anger 123

  depression 123

  grief 123

  guilt 123

  role reversal 123

  social isolation 123

an empathetic approach 83, 84

empathy 83, 103

employment 126

engagement studies 67

epidemiology 2

evaluation 43

F

Familial AD 14

early-onset 15

late-onset 15

familial relationships 125

families 59

family demands 126

feedback 68

financial abuse 76

forgetfulness 105

frustration 86

functional capacity 33

functioning

  cognitive 66

  neurological 66

G

genetic

causative factors 14

link studies 14

make-up 8

geriatric assessment 32

  annual GP 32

geriatric health nurse visito 41

geriatric nurse visitors 3, 16, 40

geriatricians 135

A global approach 52

grandiose ideas 75

guidance

  marriage 114

  sex 114

H

hallucinations 24

auditory 11

visual 11

haloperidol 102

Hamilton Depression Rating

  Scale 31

hazards 133

health 126

health visitors 3, 40, 135

HIV 13

a holistic model 47

homosexual tendencies 114

hostility 99

Huntington's disease 13

hygiene 55, 134

hypoglycaemia 13

hypothermia 134

hypothyroidism 13, 31

I

IADL

See Also Instrumental Activities of

  Daily Living

identification bracelet 106

immobility 23

impairment

  cognitive 60

  neurological 60, 62

  visual spatial 85

incidence 3

incontinence 18, 23, 40

  assessment 118

  management 118

individuality 48

infantalisation 64, 137

Inflammatory systemic disease 13

informal support 126

insomnia 110

instability 23

Instrumental Activities of Dàily

  Living 28

intervention 43

intimidation 64, 138

invalidation 64, 138

investigations 32

L

labelling 64
LBD 10
  See Also Lewy body disease
learning
  motor 53
  operant 53
  verbal 53
Lewy body type 11, 13
libido
  loss of 115, 116
life reviews 46
liver function tests 32
loneliness 104

M

magnetic resonance imaging 38
malabsorption syndrome 13
malignant social psychology 62,
  63, 66, 68
malnutrition 23
masturbation
  public 114
MEDIC ALERT 106
memory 55, 71
  clinic 76
  deficits 76
  long-term 73, 114
  loss 53, 73
  management 76, 77
  primary 72
  problems 56
  retraining 76, 77
  short-term 72, 114
memory impairment 74
  mild 74
  moderate 74
  severe 74
mental distress 100
metabolic causes 13
MID 7, 9, 10, 16
  See Also multi-infarct dementia
mild personal detractor 68
Mini-Mental State Examination 27
minor tranquilliser 107
MMSE 28, 146
  See Also Mini-Mental State
mnemonics 77

models
  activities of daily living 53
  management 53
morosis 1
MRI 38
  See Also Magnetic resonance
  imaging
multiple sclerosis 13
mutations 8, 15

N

needs
  sexual 115
nerve plaques 14
neurofibrillary tangles 15
neurofibrils 2
neurological impairment 50
nitrazepam 102
nocturnal
  confusion 24
  wakening 111
  wandering 24
The nurse's role 39, 45
nurses
  task-centred 48
nurses
  See Also primary care team
The nursing process 43, 101
  assessment 101
  global 45
  holistic 45
  management 101
  person-centred approach 45
nursing stresses 134
nutritional causes 13

O

objectification 65, 68, 138
obsessive, repetitive behavio 18
occupational therapists 42, 133, 135
organic brain disease 71
orientation 55, 78
orientation aids 81
outpacing 64, 68
overreaction 93, 98

P

Parkinson's disease 7, 11, 13
Parkinsonism 23
patient function 51

PD 11
  See Also Parkinsons disease
perception 24
perseveration 98, 102
personality50
personality changes 124
personhood 66
PET 38
  See Also positron emission
  tomography
physical abuse 101
  functioning, 53
  health 50
planning 43
Plissit Model 115
postmortem 16
potentially disruptive behavour
  agitation 95
  disinhibited toileting 95
  emotional outbursts 95
  night-time restlessness 95
  overreactions 95
  physical aggression 95
  screaming 95
  shouting 95
  uninhibited sexual behaviour95
  verbal rudeness 95
  wandering 95
practice nurse 47
premorbid personality 99
premorbid relationships 126
prevalence 2
The primary care team 135
primary cerebral degeneration13
problem behaviour 97
  management 93
problems
  emotional 123
profiles
  group 68
  individual 68
prognosis 7
props 81
provocation
  sexual 116
pseudodementia 29
psychiatrists 135
psycho-geriatric appraisal22
psychogeriatricians 135

psychometric tests 16, 36
psychomotor skills 18
psychotherapeutic care 48
  Q
  quality of life 62, 65
  R
  rating scales 27, 34, 41
  dementia 41
  depression41
reality orientation 42, 46, 78, 80,
  100
reclusiveness 109
recollection 73, 82
referral126
  psychosexual 116
Refusal of service 139
rehabilitation 76
relaxation 67
remembrance 81
reminiscence 74, 81, 82
reminiscence therapies 42
remotivation82
renal 13
respite care 82, 130
restlessness 46, 97
restraints 107
  chemical 107
  physical 107
retrieval 73
  active 73
RO 82, 85
  See also: reality orientation 80
  S
  screening tools 32
searching 104
sedation
  daytime 107
sedative 107
self-care 80
self-esteem 100
  loss of 109
self-exposure 114
self-expression 67
self-neglect 23
self-respect 67
self-worth 48, 82, 84, 137
sense of loss127
separation 105

sexual abuse 114
sexual activity 113
sexuality 55, 113, 116
  adverse features 117
shortfalls
  attention 71
  imagery 71
  language 71
  memory 71
  perception 71
  reasoning 71
silent protest 109
sleep disturbance 102
sleepiness 16
smoking 133
social interaction of communi 71
social isolation 53
social psychology 50, 62
social work departments 126
  day care 127
  home helps 127
  laundry services 127
  Meals on Wheels 127
  respite care 127
social worker 135
socialisation 80
status 66
stigmatisation 137
stress 128, 129, 139
Sundown syndrome 93, 111
support organisations 140
support systems 126
systemic lupus erythematosis 13
    T
  team leaders 40
temazepam 107
therapeutic touch 116
therapy
  reminiscence 46, 82, 83
  resolution 46

validation 46, 83, 85
thioridazine 102, 107
thyroid function tests 32
total global experience 68
toxic confusional states 31
transient loss of consciousne 11
trauma 13
treachery 63, 138
treatment
  drug 102
  psychological 102
tremor 23
True Meeting 65
tumour 32
twenty-four-hour care
  allowance 130
    U
  understanding 83
unstable mood 128
urea 32
    V
  VAD 36
  See Also vascular dementia
validation 84
violence 93
Vitamin B12 32
vitamin B12 deficien 13, 31
voluntary associations 127, 129
    W
  wandering 18, 20, 24, 46, 93,
  102, 103, 107, 118, 124
  nocturnal 104
weight loss 23
wellbeing 67
withdrawal 84, 109
  management plan 110
working memory 72, 81